THE
BREAST

ATLAS *of* TUMOR RADIOLOGY

PHILIP J. HODES, M.D., *Editor-in-Chief*

Sponsored by

THE AMERICAN COLLEGE OF RADIOLOGY

—*with the cooperation of:*

AMERICAN CANCER SOCIETY
AMERICAN ROENTGEN RAY SOCIETY
CANCER CONTROL PROGRAM, USPHS
EASTMAN KODAK COMPANY
JAMES PICKER FOUNDATION
RADIOLOGICAL SOCIETY OF NORTH AMERICA

THE
BREAST

by

DAVID M. WITTEN, M.D., M.S. IN RADIOLOGY

Consultant, Section of Roentgenology, Mayo Clinic;
Assistant Professor of Radiology, Mayo Graduate School of Medicine
(University of Minnesota), Rochester, Minn.

YEAR BOOK MEDICAL PUBLISHERS · INC.
35 EAST WACKER DRIVE, CHICAGO

Editor's Preface

In 1960, the Committee on Radiology of the National Research Council began to consider the preparation of a tumor atlas for radiology similar in concept to the Armed Forces Institute of Pathology's "Atlas of Tumor Pathology." So successfully had the latter filled a need in pathology that it seemed reasonable to establish a similar resource for radiology. Therefore a subcommittee of the Committee on Radiology was appointed to study the concept and make recommendations.

That original committee, made up of Dr. Russell H. Morgan (Chairman), Dr. Marshall H. Brucer and Dr. Eugene P. Pendergrass, reported that a need did indeed exist and recommended that something be done about it. That report was unanimously accepted by the parent committee.

Soon thereafter, there occurred a normal change of the membership of the Committee on Radiology of the Council. This was followed by a change of the "Atlas" subcommittee, which now included Dr. E. Richard King (Chairman), Dr. Leo G. Rigler and Dr. Barton R. Young. To this new subcommittee was assigned the task of finding how the "Atlas" was to be published. Numerous avenues were explored; none seemed wholly satisfactory.

With the passing of time, it became increasingly apparent that the American College of Radiology had to be brought into the picture. It had prime teaching responsibilities; it had a Commission on Education; it seemed the logical responsible agent to launch the "Atlas." Confident of the merits of this approach, the entire Committee on Radiology of the Council became involved in focusing the attention of the American College of Radiology upon the matter.* In 1964, as the result of their persuasiveness, the Board of Chancellors of the American College of Radiology named an ad hoc committee to explore and define the scholarly scope of the "Atlas" and the probable costs. In 1965, the ad hoc committee recommended that the College

---

* At that time, the Committee on Radiology included, in addition to the subcommittee, Drs. John A. Campbell, James B. Dealy, Jr., Melvin M. Figley, Hymer L. Friedell, Howard B. Latourette, Alexander Margulis, Ernest A. Mendelsohn, Charles M. Nice, Jr., and Edward W. Webster.

sponsor and publish the "Atlas." Accordingly, an Editorial Advisory Committee was chosen to work within the Commission on Education with authority to select an Editor-in-Chief. At the same time, the College provided funds for starting the project and began representations for grants-in-aid without which the "Atlas" would never be published.

No history of the "Atlas of Tumor Radiology" would be complete without specific recording of the generous response of the several radiological societies, as well as the private and Federal granting institutions whose names appear on the title page and below among our acknowledgments. It was their tangible evidence of confidence in the project that provided everyone with enthusiasm and eagerness to achieve our goal.

The "Atlas of Tumor Radiology" includes all major organ systems. It is intended to be a systematic body of pictorial and written information dealing with the roentgen manifestations of tumors. No attempt has been made to provide an atlas equivalent of a medical encyclopedia. Nevertheless the "Atlas" is designed to serve as an important reference source and teaching file for all physicians, not radiologists alone.

The twelve volumes of the "Atlas," to be completed in 1971-72, are: *The Hemopoietic and Lymphatic Systems,* by Gerald D. Dodd and Sidney Wallace; *The Bones and Joints,* by Gwilym Lodwick and Lent C. Johnson; *The Lower Respiratory Tract and Thoracic Contents,* by Roy R. Greening and J. Haynes Heslep; *The Gastrointestinal Tract,* by Arthur K. Finkelstein and George N. Stein; *The Urinary Tract,* by John A. Evans and Morton Bosniak; *The Breast,* by David M. Witten; *The Head and Neck,* by Gilbert H. Fletcher and Bao-Shan Jing; *The Nervous System and the Eye,* by Juan M. Taveras and Ernest W. Wood; *The Female Generative System,* by G. Melvin Stevens and John F. Weigen; *The Endocrines,* by Howard L. Steinbach and Hideyo Minagi; *The Accessory Digestive Organs,* by Robert E. Wise; and *The Spine,* by Bernard S. Epstein.

Some overlapping of material in several volumes is inevitable, for example, tumors of the female generative system, tumors of the endocrine glands and tumors of the urinary tract. This is considered to be an asset. It assures the specialist completeness in the volume or volumes that concern him and provides added breadth and depth of knowledge for those interested in the entire series.

The broad scope of the "Atlas of Tumor Radiology" has precluded its preparation by a single or even several authors. To maintain uniformity of format, rather rigid criteria were established early. These included manner of presentation, size of illustrations, as well as style of headings, subheadings and legends. The authors were encouraged to keep the text at a minimum, freeing as much space as possible for large illustrations and meaningful legends. The "Atlas" is to be just that, an "atlas," not a series of "texts." The authors were urged, also, to keep the bibliography brief.

The selection of suitable authors for the "Atlas" was extremely difficult, and to a degree invidious. For the final choice, the Editor-in-Chief accepts full responsibility. It is but fair to record, however, that his Editorial Advisory Committee accepted his recommendations. The format of the "Atlas," too, was the choice of the Editor-in-Chief, again with the concurrence of his advisory group. Should the "Atlas of Tumor Radiology" fall short of its goals, the fault will lie with the Editor-in-Chief alone; his Editorial Advisory Committee was selfless in its dedication to the purposes of the "Atlas," rendering invaluable advice and guidance whenever asked to do so.

As medical knowledge expands, medical concepts change. In medicine, the written word considered true today may not be so tomorrow. The text of the "Atlas," considered true today, therefore may not be true tomorrow. What may not change, what may ever remain true, may be the illustrations of the "Atlas of Tumor Radiology." Their legends may change as our conceptual levels advance. But the validity of the roentgen findings there recorded should endure. Thus, if the fidelity with which the roentgenograms have been reproduced is of superior order, the illustrations in the "Atlas" should long serve as sources for reference no matter what revisions of the text become necessary with advancing medical knowledge.

ACKNOWLEDGMENTS

The American College of Radiology, its Commission on Education, the Editorial Advisory Committee, the authors and the Editor-in-Chief wish to acknowledge their grateful appreciation:

1. For the grants-in-aid so willingly and repeatedly provided by The American Cancer Society, The American Roentgen Ray Society, The Cancer Control Program, National Center for Chronic Disease Control (USPHS Grant No. 59481), The James Picker Foundation, and The Radiological Society of North America.

2. For the superb glossy print reproductions provided by the Radiography Markets Division, Eastman Kodak Company. Special mention must be made of the sustained interest of Mr. George R. Struck, its Assistant Vice-President and General Manager. We applaud particularly Mr. William

S. Cornwell, Technical Associate and Editor Emeritus of Kodak's *Medical Radiography and Photography,* as well as his associates, Mr. Charles C. Heckman and Mr. Stanley J. Pietrzkowski and others in the Photo Service Division, whose expertise provided the "Atlas" with its incomparable photographic reproductions.

3. To Year Book Medical Publishers, for their personal involvement with and judicious guidance in the many problems of publication. There were occasions when the publisher questioned the quality of certain illustrations. Almost always the judgment of the authors and the Editor-in-Chief prevailed because of the importance of the original roentgenograms and the singular fidelity of their reproduction.

4. To the Associate Editors, particularly Mrs. Anabel I. Janssen, whose talents lightened the burden of the Editor-in-Chief and helped establish the style of presentation of the material.

5. To the Staff of the American College of Radiology, especially Messrs. William C. Stronach, Otha Linton, Keith Gundlach and William Melton, for continued conceptual and administrative efforts of unusual competence.

This volume of the "Atlas," the second of the series to be published, reflects great credit upon its author, Dr. Witten. He is to be congratulated for his care and diligence in the selection of his material. His confidence in our ability to reproduce his magnificent mammograms strained every resource at our command. Prime fidelity was the challenge; we believe it has been met in superior fashion. We are proud to add this volume of the "Atlas of Tumor Radiology" to the literature concerned with mammography.

The "Atlas of Tumor Radiology" is being published in a time when massive scientific effort is taking place at an unprecedented rate and on an unprecedented scale. We hope that our final product will provide an authoritative summary of our current knowledge of the roentgen manifestations of tumors.

PHILIP J. HODES
Editor-in-Chief

Editorial Advisory Committee

HARRY L. BERMAN	LEO G. RIGLER
VINCENT P. COLLINS	PHILIP RUBIN
E. RICHARD KING	

Author's Preface

ROENTGENOGRAPHIC EXAMINATION of the breast (mammography) was introduced in 1930 by Warren. In the ensuing decade it was studied extensively and for a time had quite a vogue. During this period, a number of investigators including among others Lockwood, Hicken, Seabold and Gershon-Cohen produced diagnostic roentgenograms and demonstrated a high diagnostic accuracy for this examination. Despite its promise, however, inherent technical and interpretive difficulties of the approach caused radiologists, surgeons and other physicians dealing with disease of the breast to view the procedure with skepticism. As a result, interest gradually declined. In the late 1940's and early 1950's interest in mammography was reawakened when Leborgne introduced an improved roentgenographic technique based on the use of an x-ray tube having a small focal spot, x-rays generated at low voltage, and fine grain film. This technique produced films of improved diagnostic quality, enabling Leborgne and subsequently Gershon-Cohen to describe the roentgenographic characteristics of most types of tumors of the breast and to demonstrate the value of mammography in clinical practice. It was Leborgne who first recognized and demonstrated the importance of granular calcifications in the diagnosis of breast cancer.

Despite the excellent results obtained by these pioneer investigators, it remained for Egan in 1960 to rekindle general interest in this examination. His excellent results coupled with his enthusiasm and courtesy in training large numbers of fellow radiologists in his technique have been instrumental in making mammography a practical, widely used clinical tool.

It appears that the contribution of mammography to the study of diseases of the breast is twofold. First, it provides a means for detection of clinically unsuspected cancer; second, and probably of greater long-range importance, it provides a new vantage point from which cancer of the breast can be studied and serves as a stimulus for investigation and development of new modalities for diagnosis of disease of the breast.

Mammography presents many special problems in roentgenographic technique and interpretation which are unique or nearly unique to this field. It is beyond the scope of this volume to present a detailed discussion of each of these points, but an attempt has been made to present the basic principles of roentgenography which bear most heavily on the successful use of this technique. The principal effort, however, has been directed toward presentation of a broad cross-section of the roentgenographic findings produced by tumors and tumor-like lesions.

Recognition of the limitations of mammography (many tumors cannot be identified on the mammogram, and roentgenographic findings often do not clearly distinguish benign from malignant disease) is essential to the successful clinical application of this technique. For this reason, many examples of confusing or equivocal lesions are included in order that the reader will be fully aware of their common occurrence and the problems of diagnosis and management that they present.

Acknowledgment must be given to Dr. Philip J. Hodes for his unstinting efforts to assure the high quality of the reproductions of radiographs and for guidance as well as much constructive advice in preparation of this volume of the Atlas. Dr. Robert D. Knapp, Jr., of the Section of Publications of the Mayo Clinic, has contributed substantially by his careful editing of the text and his many helpful suggestions.

Mr. William S. Cornwell and his associates of the Eastman Kodak Company deserve special thanks. These men have prepared all but a very few of the illustrations, and it is through their skill and dedication to excellence that superb reproductions of very difficult roentgenograms have been achieved.

DAVID M. WITTEN

THE
BREAST

CHAPTER 1

Radiography of the Breast– Basic Concepts

RADIOGRAPHIC DIAGNOSIS of tumors of the breast has evolved in a decade from an obscure, rarely practiced, investigative procedure into a useful and practical clinical tool. The revival of interest in this examination is the direct result of the development of improved radiographic techniques for study of the soft tissues of the breast and the subsequent demonstration that breast disease and especially cancer can be diagnosed when it is not suspected from physical examination alone.

Mammography, as plain-film radiography of the breast usually is called, is a specialized soft tissue type of radiographic technique. It is only one among a variety of techniques which have been devised for study of tumors of the breast (others include radiopaque contrast study of the mammary ducts, xeroradiography, angiography, lymphangiography and thermography), but it is the only technique which has gained widespread acceptance in clinical practice, and for this reason is the only technique to be considered in detail in this volume.

SOFT-TISSUE RADIOGRAPHY.—The term soft-tissue radiography is used to describe a radiographic technique designed specifically for study of the anatomic and pathologic characteristics of soft tissues. It differs from conventional radiography in at least three important respects: (1) X-rays generated at very low voltage (20–35 kvp as contrasted to the 60–120 kvp commonly used in radiography) are used to make the films. (2) Special fine-grain x-ray films of the "industrial" type, which have both high inherent contrast and high resolution, are used to depict soft tissue anatomic details which range downward in size to the limits of visibility. (3) No contrast medium is injected into either the ductal system or the breast parenchyma to demonstrate disease.

For detailed discussion of the techniques of mammography, the reader is referred to the works of Egan,[1] Gershon-Cohen,[2] Kirka,[3] Stanton and Lightfoot[4] and Siler and associates.[5]

Characteristically, radiographs made with x-rays generated in the 20–35 kvp range show the fatty tissues in the breast in sharp contrast to the non-fatty tissues such as mammary ducts, fibrous tissue, skin and tumor tissue. The explanation for this phenomenon lies in the fact that at these low kilovoltage ranges, fat absorbs relatively fewer x-rays and is therefore less radiopaque than the other tissues in the breast. (Physicists frequently refer to this as *differential absorption*.) Since fatty tissue is present throughout the breast and is the predominant tissue in the majority of patients in the cancer age group as well as in many individuals during the early reproductive years, it is possible to visualize abnormal tissues and patterns of tissue growth, which identify and differentiate the various benign and malignant diseases indigenous to the breast.

MAMMOGRAPHIC VIEWS.—Conventional mammographic technique requires two views of each breast and one view of each axilla. The craniocaudad view (Fig. **1**) and the mediolateral view (Fig. **2**) demonstrate the major portion of the breast and, since they are made at right angles to one another, permit accurate localization of any lesion in the breast. The axillary view (Fig. **3**) is used for study of the axillary tail and for demonstration of axillary lymph nodes.

In addition to the three standard views of the breast, several types of special views have been devised. The most important are spot films to show localized regions of the breast with greater clarity and films made during compression of the breast to immobilize and flatten the tissue in order to enhance detail and to increase uniformity of exposure (Fig. **4**). For the craniocaudad view, special curved films which are cut to fit the contour of the chest wall are occasionally very helpful for demonstrating lesions which lie close to the chest wall or at the extreme edges of the breast. Films made with the breast in a dependent position and films made with the breast immersed in oil or water have been used by some but never have been generally accepted as practical or particularly useful in diagnosis.

DIAGNOSTIC ACCURACY.—Mammograms of the highest technical quality and interpretation of the films by a radiologist experienced with this technique are requisites to successful mammography. If either of these elements

---

[1] Egan, R. L.: *Mammography* (Springfield, Ill.: Charles C Thomas, Publisher, 1964).
[2] Gershon-Cohen, J.: Am. J. Roentgenol. 84:224, 1960.
[3] Kirka, C.: Cathode Press 19:32, 1962.
[4] Stanton, L., and Lightfoot, D. A.: Radiology 83:442, 1964.
[5] Siler, W. M., *et al.*: Am. J. Roentgenol. 91:910, 1964.

TABLE 1.—DIAGNOSTIC ACCURACY OF MAMMOGRAPHY

AUTHORS	CASES	HISTOPATHOLOGIC DIAGNOSIS					
		Benign Radiographic Diagnosis			Malignant Radiographic Diagnosis		
		Malig., %	Benign, %	Uncertain, %	Malig., %	Benign, %	Uncertain, %
Clark et al.*	1,580	10	90	—	79	21	—
Egan†	1,217	9	91	—	97	3	—
Friedman et al.‡	776	9	75	16	68	18	13
Ingleby and Gershon-Cohen§	536	0.5	65	35	63	3	34
Wolfe‖	759	12	88	—	92	8	—

* Clark, R. L., et al.: Am. J. Surg. 109:127, 1965.
† Egan, R. L.: Mammography (Springfield, Ill.: Charles C Thomas, Publisher, 1964).
‡ Friedman, A. K., et al.: Radiology 86:886, 1966.
§ Ingleby, H., and Gershon-Cohen, J.: Comparative Anatomy, Pathology, and Roentgenology of the Breast (Philadelphia: University of Pennsylvania Press, 1960).
‖ Wolfe, J. N.: Radiology 83:244, 1964.

is missing, diagnostic accuracy is poor. If both are present, the large majority of both malignant and benign tumors of the breast can be identified and correctly diagnosed preoperatively. The reported accuracy of diagnosis in most large series ranges from about 70 to 85%, and in exceptional circumstances, in excess of 90% of these lesions can be identified (Table 1).

It must be emphasized that not all malignant lesions can be demonstrated by mammography (up to 20% were not seen in some series) and that differentiation of benign disease from malignant disease on the basis of radiographic characteristics is often not clear-cut.

A number of factors in addition to the technical quality of films affect diagnostic accuracy. Among these, the location of the lesion and its radiographic appearance are important though not the major causes of diagnostic errors. For example, a mass located at the periphery of the breast may not be included on the films, or carcinoma may mimic benign disease in appearance; in either case, the lesion will be incorrectly diagnosed. The radiographic density of the breast has a greater influence on diagnostic accuracy than either of these, however. As was pointed out earlier, in the fatty breast, lesions are well demonstrated; but in the radiographically dense breast, where fat content is low, tumors are badly obscured and difficult to identify. Accuracy in the diagnosis of carcinoma is about 50% for premenopausal patients with dense breasts but frequently exceeds 90% for postmenopausal patients with fatty breasts (Table 2).

CLINICAL CONCEPTS.—Mammography, like radiography of other organs, is not meant to replace conventional clinical methods for detection and evaluation of disease of the breast; rather, its purpose is to supply information which cannot be gained from physical examination alone.

TABLE 2.—RELATION OF RADIOLOGIC INTERPRETATION TO HISTOPATHOLOGIC DIAGNOSIS ACCORDING TO AGE OF PATIENTS

	HISTOPATHOLOGIC DIAGNOSIS					
	Nonmalignant			Malignant		
	Radiographic Diagnosis		True Neg.	Radiographic Diagnosis		True Pos.
AGE, YR.	Nonmalig.	Malig.	Rate, %*	Nonmalig.	Malig.	Rate, %†
Less than 30	240	3	97.2	4	4	50.0
30–44	440	23	94.9	28	35	55.6
45–59	235	45	84.5	44	147	77.0
60 and older	74	35	67.9	20	187	90.3

* True negative rate is percentage of nonmalignant lesions correctly interpreted as nonmalignant on mammogram.
† True positive rate is percentage of cancers correctly diagnosed by mammography. (Modified from Clark, R. L., et al.: Am. J. Surg. 109:127, 1965.)

Its primary goal is detection of occult or clinically unsuspected cancer; but beyond this, it has proved useful for study of the symptomatic but clinically normal breast, for preoperative assessment of the nature and extent of disease of a patient with palpable lesions in the breast, and as a screening examination for cancer detection, especially for patients who are at high risk for developing cancer.

The presence of a palpable dominant mass or of a number of masses in one or both breasts necessitates prompt biopsy and histologic examination of tissue. In such cases, the mammogram serves to confirm the physical findings and at the same time provides additional information on the nature and extent of the disease process, which aids both the surgeon and the operating room personnel in planning for the operation. In some instances, mammography may help avoid the delay in treatment of carcinoma which results from the common practice of waiting through one to two menstrual cycles to see if the nodule decreases in size; and it may reveal the presence of associated, yet clinically unsuspected, carcinoma in the same or opposite breast. Mammography does not alter the conventional clinical indications for biopsy, but rather adds to them.

Women with breast symptoms (such as localized pain or tenderness) and signs (such as nipple retraction, generalized nodularity of the parenchyma and bilateral serous discharge from the nipples) are not ordinarily candidates for biopsy if no discrete lesion is palpable in the breast. However, a degree of uncertainty is always present in the diagnosis and management of these patients, and mammography provides an alternative method for detecting disease if it is present. If no evidence of carcinoma or other significant lesion is seen, the mammogram confirms the clinical impression that no operable lesion is present and at the same time gives added assurance to the surgeon planning conservative management of the patient.

Routine mammography of asymptomatic patients with no breast complaints and no evidence of a lesion in the breast on physical examination has been advocated as a screening examination for detection of early cancer. Screening is most productive and, in fact, is clearly a valuable adjunct to the physical examination for patients who are at high risk for development of cancer, for example, the woman with a strong family history of cancer of the breast or the woman who has had one breast removed because of carcinoma. Early carcinoma of clinically normal women who are *not* in high-risk groups can be detected, but it is not clear that the yield of carcinoma in these cases is adequate to justify the expense in time and effort required for the screening of large numbers of patients or that mammographic screening can substantially improve survival rates associated with malignant disease of the breast.

It is important for all physicians who use mammography to recognize that, while it does supply important diagnostic information, it does not replace the physical examination nor alter the established clinical criteria for biopsy. Because some carcinomas mimic benign disease in appearance and others are not adequately demonstrated by mammography, a clinically suspect lesion should be biopsied even if the mammogram suggests that it is benign; conversely, since benign disease can mimic carcinoma in its radiographic appearance, a mastectomy should never be performed on the basis of a mammographic diagnosis of carcinoma without prior biopsy and histologic proof of the malignant character of the lesion.

Figure 1.—Technique: craniocaudad view.

A, position of patient: Seated comfortably with the shoulder (**a**) drawn back slightly and relaxed. The head is turned to the side opposite the breast to be examined. The breast is rested directly on the film holder (**b**) and is supported by a stand which can be adjusted to the proper height. (Skin folds caused by improper support and positioning of the breast must be avoided.) The nipple (**c**) must be in profile and the x-ray beam centered at the base of the breast in the midline (**d**), at the junction of the breast and the chest wall.

B, mammogram: Body of the breast in the superior-inferior projection. Note that the anterior portion of the breast is demonstrated but that tissue lying close to the chest wall or in the axillary extension of the breast cannot be projected on the film.

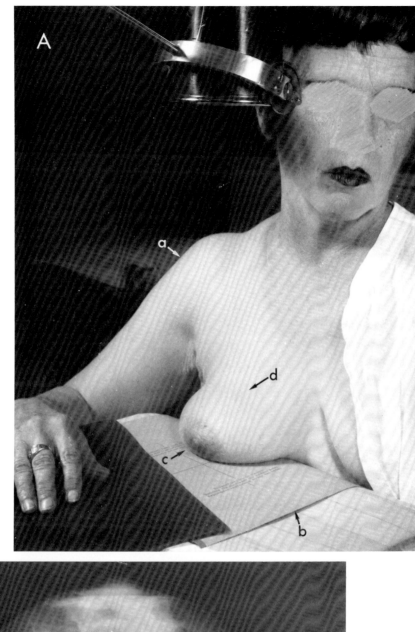

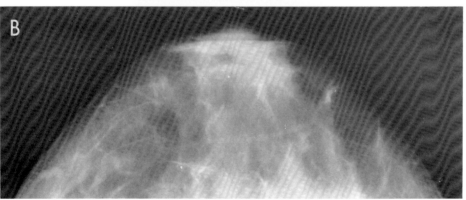

Figure 1 · Technique: Craniocaudad View / 7

Figure 2.—Technique: mediolateral view.

A, position of the patient: Lying on her side in a comfortable relaxed position with the arm on the side of the breast to be examined raised above the head. The breast rests on the film holder which is supported by sandbags and is bent slightly (**a**) to conform to the contour of the breast. The patient gently retracts the opposite breast with her free hand (**b**) to prevent its obscuring the breast under study. The nipple (**c**) is in profile. The x-ray beam is centered on the midline of the breast where it joins the chest wall (**d**).

As in the craniocaudad view (Fig. **1**), one must take care to have the nipple in profile and to avoid skin folds or other distortions of the breast caused by improper support or positioning.

B, mammogram: Entire breast in mediolateral projection. When the patient has been properly positioned, this view shows the retromammary space (**d**), the breast tissues close to the chest wall (**e**) which are not included on the craniocaudad view and the axillary extension or tail of the breast (**f**) as well as of the tissues in the anterior part of the breast. Since this view is made at right angles to the craniocaudad view, one may localize any lesion present in both views.

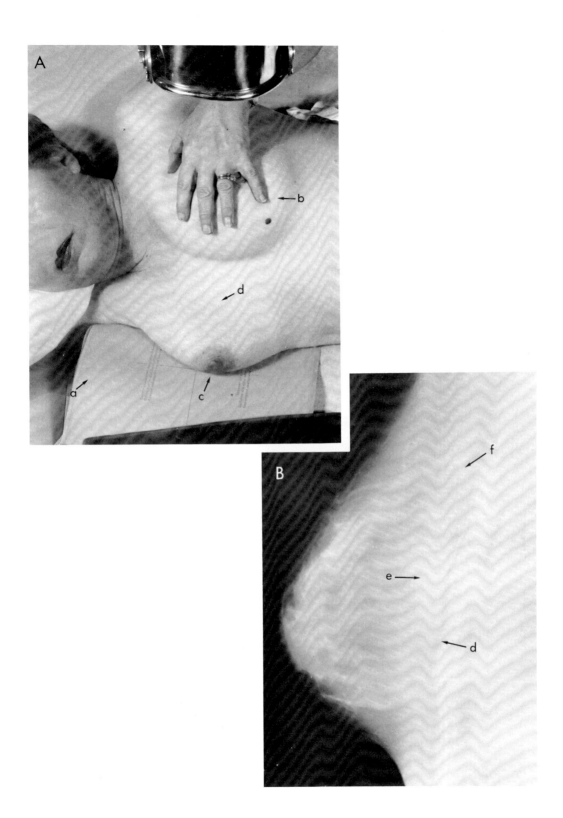

Figure 2 · Technique: Mediolateral View / 9

Figure 3.—Technique: axillary view.

A, position of patient: Lying on her back in a recumbent position but rotated 15–30° from the supine. The arm on the side of the breast to be examined (**a**) is abducted to 90°. (This position prevents the scapula from overlying and obscuring the axillary tissues.) The film holder is centered under the axilla with its upper edge even with the top of the shoulder (**b**) and the midline of the film (**c**) parallel to the chest wall. The x-ray beam is centered about 5 cm below the axillary fold (**d**), in line with the edge of the chest wall.

B, mammogram: Demonstration of the axillary extension of the breast (**e**) and the axillary lymph nodes if they are enlarged.

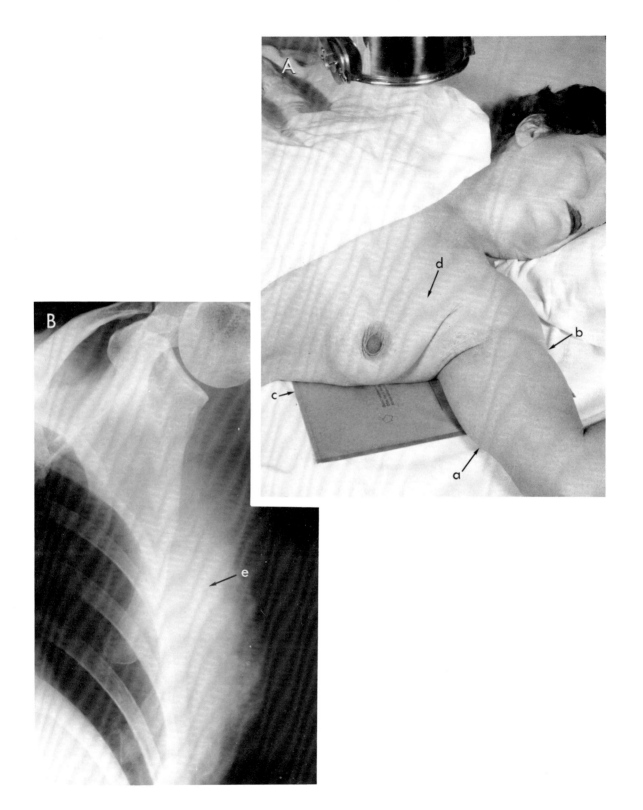

Figure 3 · Technique: Axillary View / 11

Figure 4.—Technique: compression spot film.

Position of patient is the same as for either the craniocaudad or the mediolateral projection. Spot films of the breast can be made with or without compression. Such films of localized regions of the breast are frequently of assistance in demonstrating anatomic details which are obscured or poorly demonstrated on films of the entire breast.

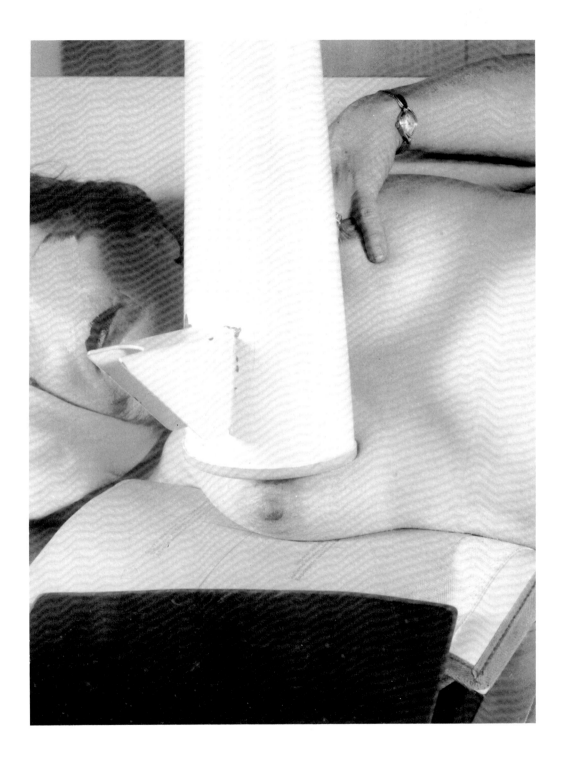

Figure 4 · Technique: Compression Spot Film / 13

CHAPTER 2

The Normal Breast

THE RADIOGRAPHIC APPEARANCE of the normal breast varies from patient to patient, depending on such factors as age, hormonal status and the relative proportion of fatty tissue to nonfatty tissue; but the basic details of anatomy which are important to diagnosis are constant and can be identified and evaluated on any mammogram of satisfactory technical quality.

ANATOMIC FEATURES

The principal anatomic features seen on the mammogram (see Fig. **5**) are the cutaneous structures, including the skin, areola and nipple; the body of the breast (corpus mammae), including its axillary extension; the subcutaneous fat; the retromammary space, and the mammary veins. Neither the lymphatics nor the axillary lymph nodes are seen on mammograms of normal patients.

BODY OF THE BREAST (CORPUS MAMMAE).—The body of the breast is contained within the superficial and deep layers of the superficial fascia of the anterior chest wall. It is composed of the glandular tissues of the breast along with fibrous connective tissue and fat which support them.

Within the glandular portions of the breast, 15–20 separate branching ducts are found. Each forms a separate anatomic unit, known as a lobe, which empties onto the nipple through a single lactiferous duct (see Fig. **6**). Deep to the nipple (**a**) and beneath the areola, a dilated portion of the lactiferous duct known as the *ampulla* or *lactiferous sinus* (**b**) is found. Beyond this point, the duct branches repeatedly to form multiple *lobules* (**c**), each of which is formed from clusters of *alveoli* (**d**) communicating with the small branches of the lactiferous duct.

Connective tissue septa in the form of loosely defined bundles and partitions bind together and separate the glandular portions of the breast. Some attach to the dermis of the skin. The larger of these form the *suspensory* (Cooper's) *ligaments* of the breast (see Fig. **6**). Interspersed throughout the connective tissue stroma are deposits of fat which contribute substantially to the contour of the breast and determine to a large degree its radiolucency.

On the mammogram (Fig. **7**), the details of glandular anatomy just described are seen only in part. The large lactiferous ducts and the lactiferous sinuses deep to the nipple can be identified as discrete cordlike structures in some instances, but more commonly the lactiferous ducts form an ill-defined linear pattern of density which converges on the nipple. The small ducts and the alveoli along with their supporting connective tissues are seen only as irregular or patchy areas of radiopacity with no specific anatomic form. In breasts that are mainly glandular with little contrasting fatty tissue, the corpus mammae forms an irregularly radiopaque cone-shaped mass. In others, in which fatty tissue predominates, little evidence of glandular tissue is seen.

CUTANEOUS STRUCTURES.—The *skin* is of uniform thickness over the entire breast. Typically, it measures from 0.5 to 1.5 mm thick on mammograms of normal women (Fig. **8**), average about 1 mm. An increase in apparent thickness is often seen at both the areola and the inferior mammary fold where the breast joins the chest wall. This appearance is caused by sharp angulation or folding of the skin at these sites. Care must be taken to distinguish this appearance from that of true skin thickening due to disease. In many instances, normal indentations of the skin around hair follicles can be clearly seen.

The *areola* is the pigmented area surrounding the nipple. It is often wrinkled or roughened by the papillae of the areolar glands (glands of Montgomery). The areola may be visible on the mammogram as a distinct area of thickened skin; sometimes, however, it is not visible as a discrete anatomic structure.

The *nipples* may be erect (Fig. **8, A**), flattened (**8, B**) or inverted (**8, C**), in the normal state, although inversion often is associated with disease. The skin of the nipple tends to be folded or wrinkled like that of the areola. It is important to compare the appearance of the nipples of the two breasts in order that minimal amounts of thickening or retraction due to carcinoma or other disease can be detected.

SUBCUTANEOUS FAT.—A layer of fat and loose fibrous connective tissue invests the glandular portion of the breast, separating it from the skin anteriorly and the deep fascia and muscles of the chest wall posteriorly. This layer, which is recognized on the mammogram as the subcutaneous fat anteriorly and as the retromammary space posteriorly, forms an important radiologic landmark.

The layer of subcutaneous fat (Fig. **9**) separating the skin from the glandular portions of the breast varies in both thickness and prominence from individual to individual. In most instances when the body of the breast is highly glandular or when there is extensive benign disease, the subcutaneous fat forms an easily identified band of lucency which may vary in thickness from roughly 0.5 cm to 2.5 cm or more. Its thickness is not uniform and beneath the nipple it is not present, as the entire nipple region is normally occupied by radiopaque lactiferous ducts and periductal fibrous connective tissue. Large superficial veins lie within the layer of superficial fat and are easily seen. The suspensory (Cooper's) ligaments traverse the subcutaneous fat and are recognized on mammograms of some but not all women as fine strands of dense tissue extending from the body of the breast to the skin.

RETROMAMMARY SPACE.—When the patient has been properly positioned for the mediolateral projection, the retromammary space (Fig. **10**) appears as a thin line of lucency separating the body of the breast from the chest wall. It is formed of fat and loose areolar tissue lying between the deep layer of the superficial fascia and the pectoral fascia. In breasts with dense parenchyma, it rarely exceeds 0.5 cm in thickness, and it cannot be identified in fatty breasts. The importance of the retromammary space is twofold: (1) When clearly seen on the mediolateral projection, it indicates that the positioning of the patient is correct so that little if any of the breast is obscured by the chest wall. (2) In the presence of carcinoma, obliteration of the retromammary space by the tumor indicates invasion of the chest wall.

MAMMARY BLOOD VESSELS.—Of the vascular supply to the breast, only the large mammary veins can be identified on mammograms of normal patients (Fig. **11**). Most of these veins lie in the subcutaneous fat, but some deeper veins are occasionally seen. The size and distribution of the veins vary widely from individual to individual, but they tend to be symmetrical in the two breasts of the same individual. The arteries ordinarily are not seen. Their small size and pulsatile motion combine to prevent their demonstration on the mammogram. In the presence of arteriosclerosis with heavy arterial calcification, however, they are visible, and it is common to observe small calcified arteries in elderly patients.

VARIATIONS IN NORMAL RADIOGRAPHIC APPEARANCE

As pointed out previously, the radiographic appearance of the normal breast depends to a large degree on the relative proportion of fat to glandular and fibrous tissues. In the adolescent and the young sexually mature

TABLE 3.—RELATION OF TYPE OF BREAST TO AGE: 282 CONSECUTIVE
PATIENTS WITH CLINICALLY NORMAL BREASTS

		TYPE OF BREAST, % (NO.) OF CASES			
AGE, YR.	CASES	DIFFUSELY GLANDULAR	PREDOMINANTLY GLANDULAR	PREDOMINANTLY FATTY	FATTY
25	3	33(1)	67(2)	0(0)	0(0)
26–35	14	36(5)	57(8)	7(1)	0(0)
36–45	52	31(16)	48(25)	10(5)	12(6)
46–55	79	18(14)	33(26)	10(8)	39(31)
56–65	76	7(5)	32(24)	11(8)	51(39)
66–75	48	0(0)	15(7)	19(9)	67(32)
76 and older	10	0(0)	0(0)	30(3)	70(7)

woman, the glandular parenchyma and its connective tissue stroma predominate (Figs. 12 and 13), with the result that the breasts tend to be relatively radiopaque. The fat content of the breast tends to increase both with age and following pregnancy (Fig. 14). As the end of the child-bearing period approaches, involution of these hormonally dependent tissues occurs and there is replacement by fat (Figs. 15 and 16). Consequently, the breasts of most women are radiolucent after the menopause (Figs. 17 and 18) and contain little if any recognizable glandular tissue (Table 3).

Wide variation in the relative proportions of fat to glandular tissue is found from individual to individual in all age groups, however; and breasts which are predominantly fatty are not uncommon in young women, while dense, glandular breasts are frequently seen in women past the menopause.

The fact that radiographically dense breast parenchyma predominates in premenopausal patients reduces the accuracy and consequently the value of mammography for such patients. Conversely, the predominance of radiolucent fatty breasts in postmenopausal patients facilitates the identification of disease and makes the mammogram relatively more valuable as a diagnostic tool.

VARIATIONS WITH MENSTRUAL STATE AND PREGNANCY.—Despite the marked cyclic changes that occur in the breast in association with menstruation, little if any identifiable alteration in the appearance of the parenchyma of the breast is seen on mammograms made at various times during the menstrual cycle. Apparently neither the fluid engorgement of the breast nor the changes which occur in the glandular epithelium are of great enough magnitude to be visible.

During pregnancy, however, there is a marked increase in both the size of the breast and its radiographic density (Figs. 19 and 20). These changes, which first appear in the first to second month, are produced by the growth of the ductal system and the development of secretory alveoli. A marked enlargement of the mammary veins accompanies the growth of the duct system, reflecting the increased blood flow to the breast.

Figure 5.—Radiographic anatomy of normal breast.

Composite representation of the normal radiographic anatomy of the breast as seen in the mediolateral view: **a,** skin; **b,** areola; **c,** nipple; **d,** subcutaneous fat; **e,** body of the breast; **f,** axillary extension (tail) of the breast; **g,** retromammary space; **h,** veins; **i,** suspensory (Cooper's) ligaments; **j,** inferior mammary fold.

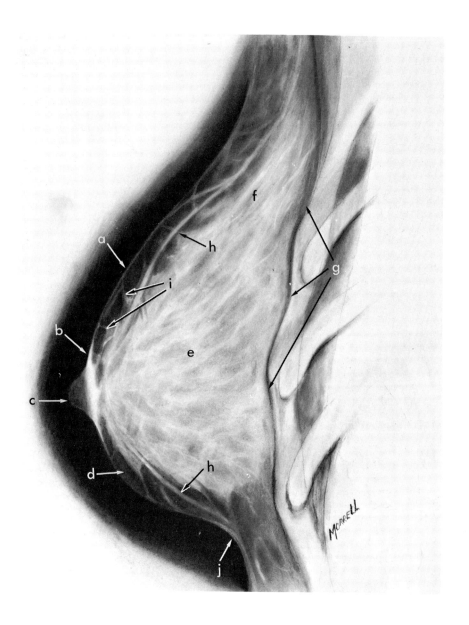

Figure 6.—Schematic diagram of mammary duct system.

A single lobe is composed of a lactiferous duct (**a**), an ampulla (**b**) and numerous lobules (**c**) made up of clusters of alveoli (**d**).

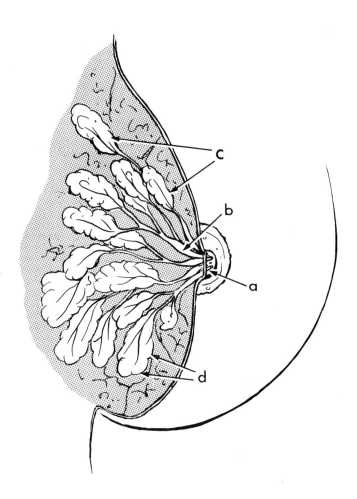

Figure 6 · **Diagram of Mammary Duct System** / **19**

Figure 7.—Body of breast (corpus mammae) of a normal 25-year-old nulliparous woman.

A, mediolateral view: **a,** body of breast; **b,** axillary extension; **c,** subcutaneous fat; **d,** retromammary space.

B, craniocaudal view: **a,** body of the breast; **c,** subcutaneous fat; **e,** veins.

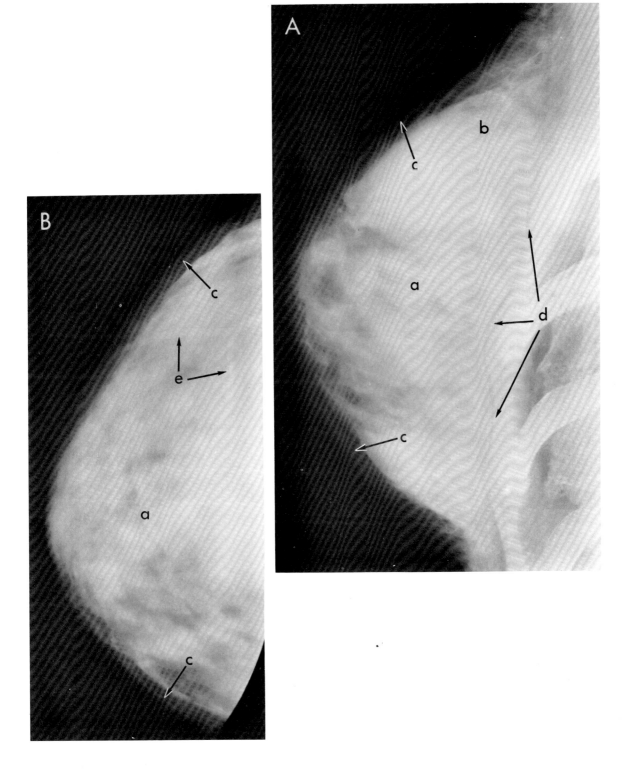

Figure 7 · Body of Breast of Nullipara / 21

Figure 8.—Cutaneous structures.

    A, lightly exposed mammogram, showing normal cutaneous structures: **a,** skin; **b,** areola; **c,** erect nipple; **d,** inferior mammary fold.

    B, normal breast with flattened nipple (**arrow**).

    C, normal breast with inverted nipple (**arrow**).

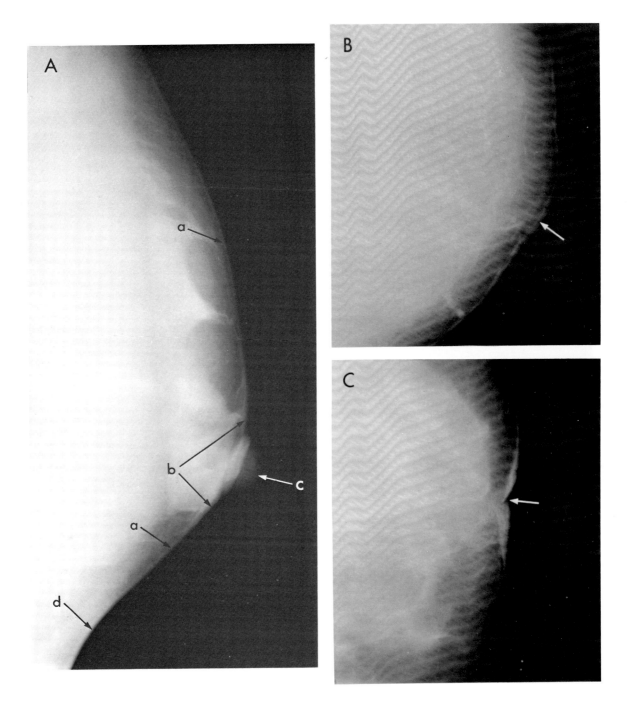

Figure 8 · Cutaneous Structures / 23

Figure 9.—Subcutaneous fat in breast of a 49-year-old woman with dense breast parenchyma.

Craniocaudal view: In the region beneath the nipple (**b**), no subcutaneous fat is seen as at (**a**). Large superficial veins (**c**) are evident within the fatty layer.

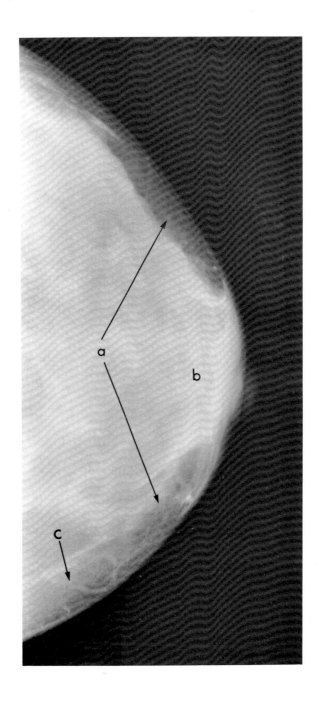

Figure 9 · Subcutaneous Fat, Dense Parenchyma / 25

Figure 10.—Retromammary space in breast of a 15-year-old girl.

Mediolateral view: Retromammary space (**a**) separates the chest wall (**b**) from the body of the breast (**c**). The breast parenchyma is dense.

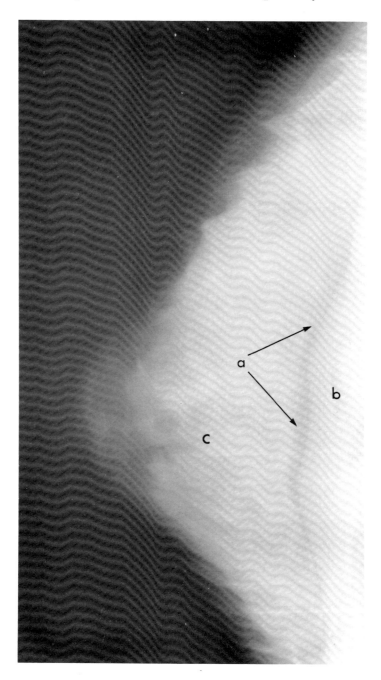

Figure 11.—Blood vessels of fatty breast of an 81-year-old woman.

Veins (**a**) and calcified arteries (**b**) are visible.

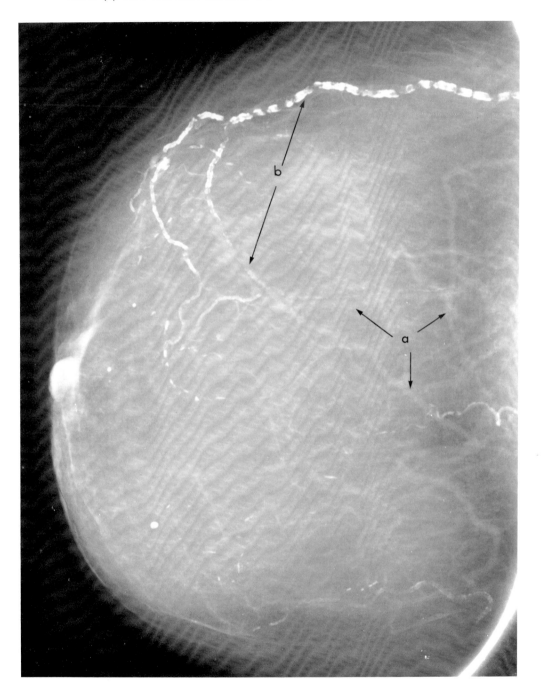

Figure 11 · Blood Vessels of Fatty Breast / 27

Figure 12.—Diffuse opacity of breast of a 15-year-old girl.

Craniocaudal view: Typical diffuse opacity of the parenchyma of the breast during adolescence, which produces a ground-glass appearance. Little fat is present. Discrete glandular structures cannot be identified in the body of the breast, and tumors such as fibroadenomas usually are obscured.

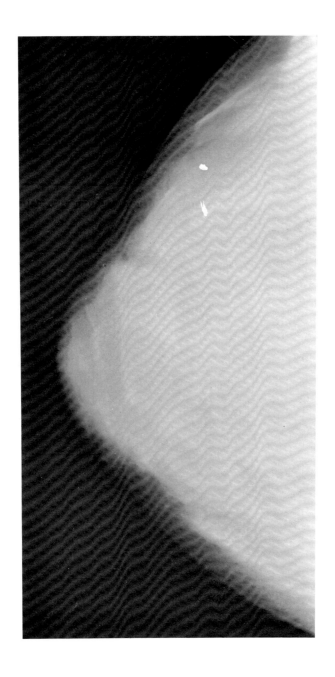

Figure 12 · Diffuse Opacity in Adolescent / 29

Figure 13.—Diffusely glandular breast of a 24-year-old nulliparous patient with no complaints relative to the breast.

A, mediolateral view.

B, craniocaudal view.

The parenchyma is dense, although it lacks the ground-glass appearance of the breast in adolescence (see Fig. **12**). Subcutaneous fat is scant, but small deposits of fat produce lucencies (**a**) throughout the body of the breast. The density of the glandular tissue is so great in this type of breast that mass lesions such as fibroadenomas are difficult to identify.

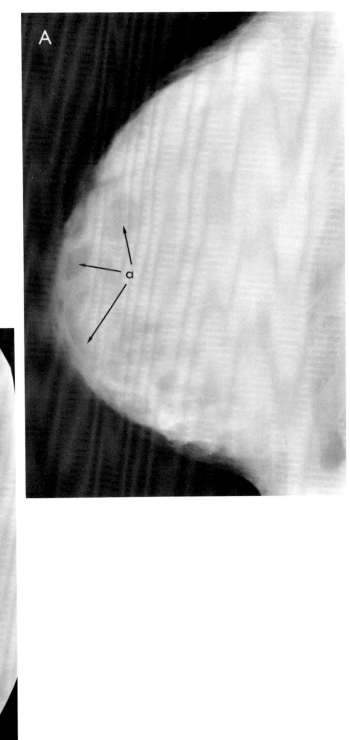

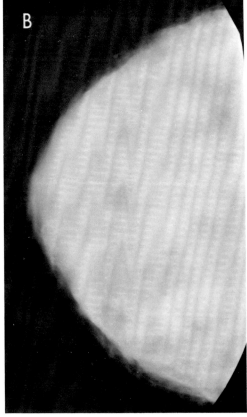

Figure 13 · Diffusely Glandular Breast in Nullipara / 31

Figure 14.—Predominantly fatty breast of a 25-year-old woman with one child.

A, mediolateral view.

B, craniocaudal view.

In the usual case, there is considerable fatty replacement of breast parenchyma after pregnancy. The glandular and fibrous tissues (**a**) are widely separated by lucent deposits of fat and appear as irregular patches and strands of tissue which tend to be oriented in the direction of the nipple (**b**).

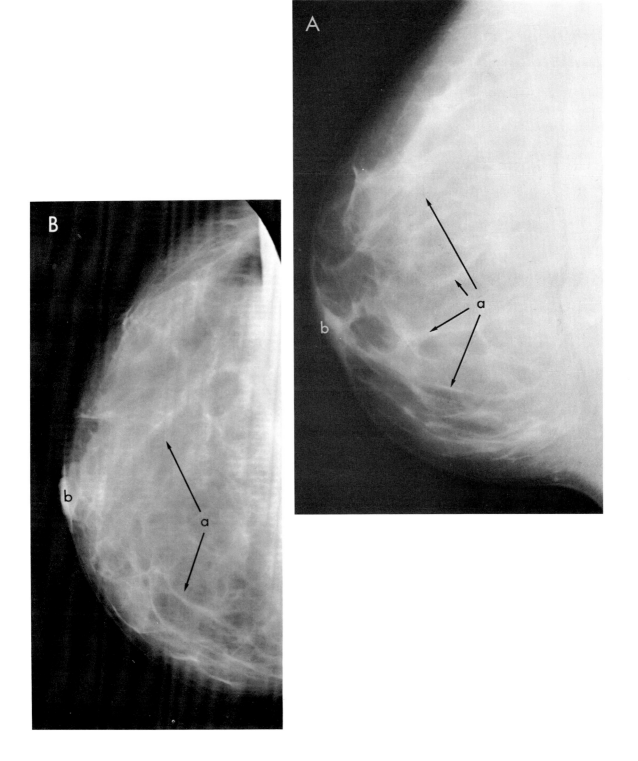

Figure 14 · Fatty Breast after Pregnancy / 33

Figure 15.—Predominantly fatty breast of a 35-year-old woman with three children.

A wide variation in the amount and distribution of glandular tissue is seen in the breasts of patients in this age group. In an average case, such as that illustrated, fat (**a**) has replaced glandular tissue to a large extent, and strands of fibrous connective tissue (**b**) are prominent.

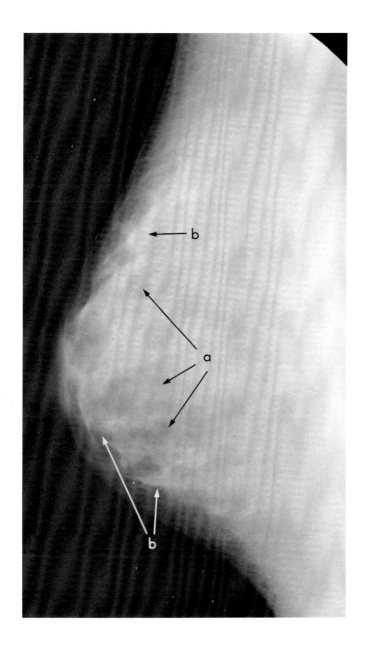

Figure 15 · Fatty Breast in Multipara / 35

Figure 16.—Predominantly fatty premenopausal breast of a 48-year-old woman.

As the menopause approaches, both the glandular parenchyma and the fibrous connective tissue stroma (**a**) involute and are replaced by fat (**b**). Fatty replacement often does not proceed at a uniform pace throughout the breast but tends to advance more rapidly close to the chest wall and in the lower half of the breast.

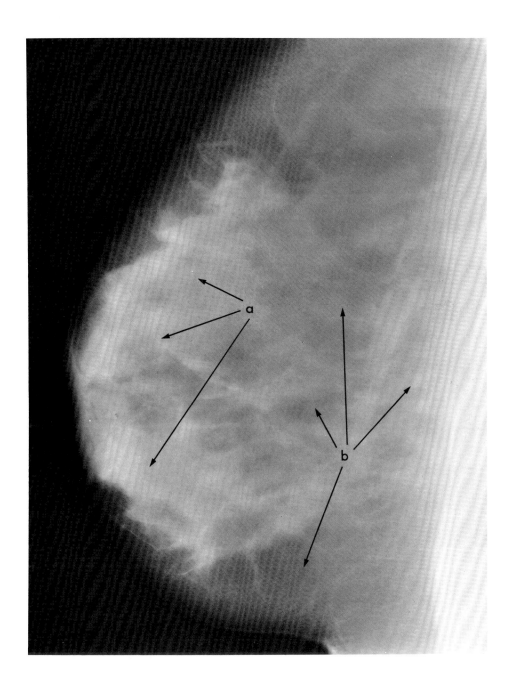

Figure 16 · Fatty Premenopausal Breast / 37

Figure 17.—Postmenopausal breast of a 61-year-old woman eight years after the last menstrual period.

A, mediolateral view.

B, craniocaudal view.

Residual radiopaque glandular and fibrous tissue (**a**) is present beneath the nipple (**b**) in the central portion of the breast and in the upper outer quadrant. Glandular tissue often persists after the menopause (see Table 3, p. 17), but in many such cases diffuse benign disease is present.

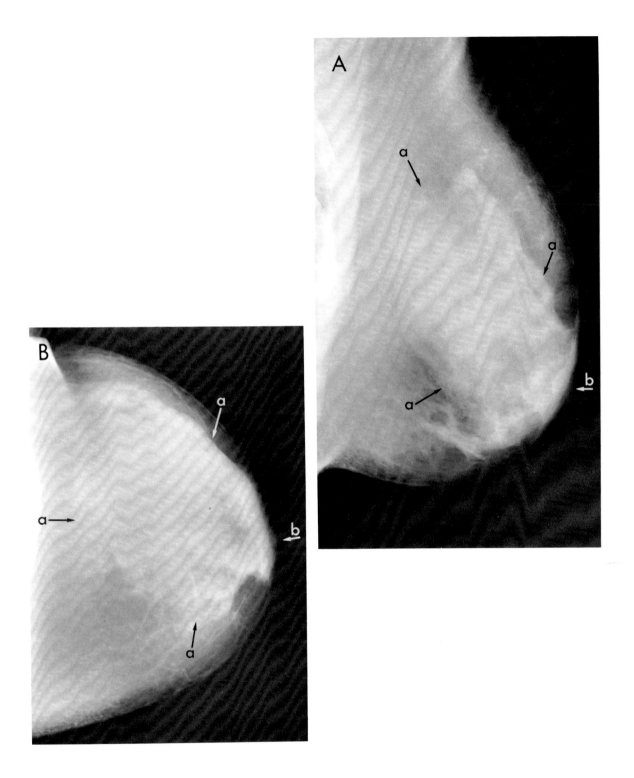

Figure 17 · Postmenopausal Breast / 39

Figure 18.—Postmenopausal breast of a 69-year-old woman.

The breast is large and the breast parenchyma has disappeared almost completely and has been replaced by fat. A few fine strands of fibrous connective tissue (**a**) persist, and the veins are prominent (**b**). Carcinoma is easily identified when present in fatty breasts. The predominance of this type in postmenopausal women accounts for the high rate of accuracy of mammography for patients in this older age group.

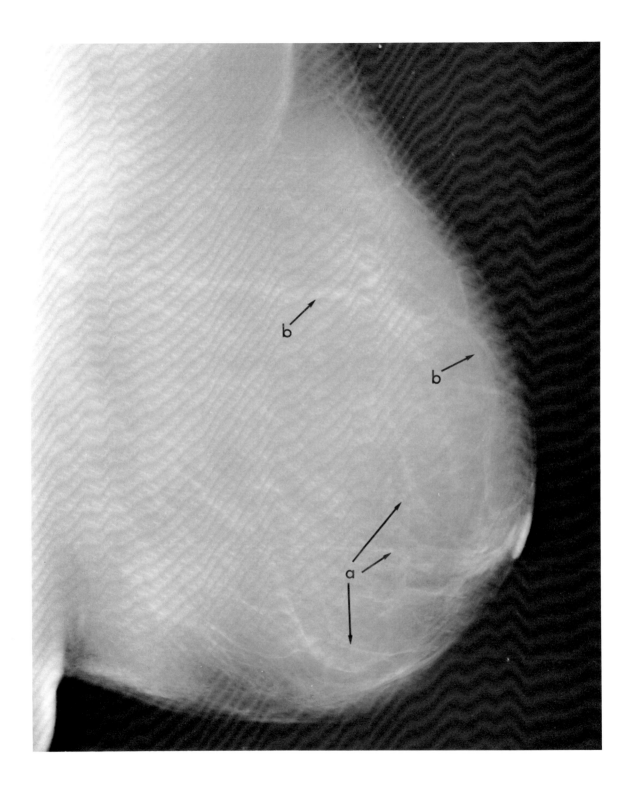

Figure 18 · Postmenopausal Breast / 41

Figure 19.—Changes in the breast during pregnancy.

A, normal, predominantly fatty breast of a nonpregnant 38-year-old woman. The glandular tissues (**a**) are sparse and the veins (**b**) are small.

B, the same patient one year later during the fourth month of pregnancy. The breast has increased in size, and there has been a marked increase in the amount and density of the glandular tissues (**a**). The veins (**b**) have doubled in size, indicating an increased flow of blood.

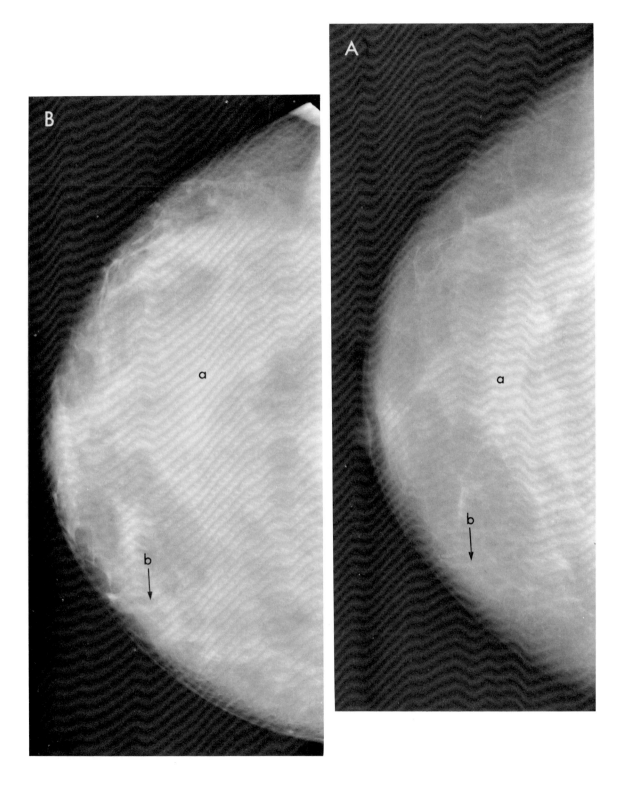

Figure 19 · Changes in Early Pregnancy / 43

Figure 20.—Breast in advanced pregnancy.

The breast of a 28-year-old woman in the seventh month of pregnancy shows the breast parenchyma (**a**) to be extremely dense; little fat remains. When carcinoma develops during pregnancy, it usually is obscured by dense overlying parenchyma and cannot be diagnosed on the mammogram until it is in an advanced stage of growth (see Chap. 4).

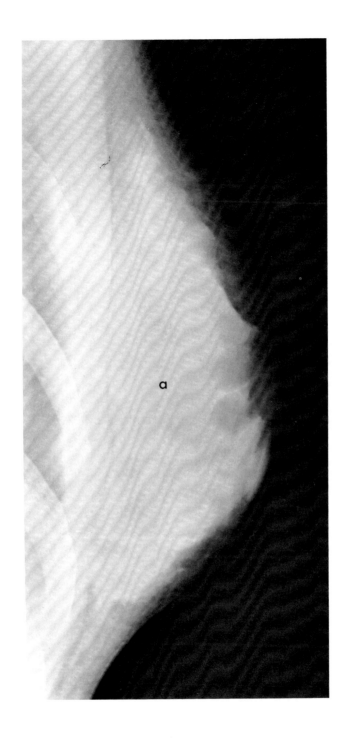

Figure 20 · Changes in Advanced Pregnancy / 45

CHAPTER 3

Benign Diseases of the Breast

BENIGN DISEASES of the breast comprise a diverse, poorly understood group of abnormalities which present widely varying radiographic appearances. Pathologically, these lesions range from diffuse bilateral alterations in the stromal and glandular components of the breast, resulting from distortion and exaggeration of the cyclic breast changes seen during the menstrual cycle, to solitary or discrete lesions which appear to arise in otherwise normal breast tissue. Two or more types of benign disease are commonly present in the same breast. In such circumstances, classification from both a morphologic and a radiographic standpoint is usually based on the dominant abnormality.

Most of the discrete benign lesions, for example, fibroadenoma and localized cyst, present well-defined and distinctive radiographic appearances which reflect the gross pathologic characteristics of the lesion. But among the diffuse benign diseases, radiographic characteristics tend to be non-specific and difficult to describe. In many cases, the radiographic appearance of diffuse benign disease is so like that of normal breast tissue that the two cannot be separated with certainty. In their advanced stages, however, and particularly when one morphologic type of abnormality dominates, characteristic radiographic patterns can be recognized.

It is of particular interest that, while the majority have radiographic characteristics which distinguish them from cancer, some benign lesions mimic cancer in almost every radiographic particular. In this presentation on benign disease, many of these confusing lesions are illustrated in order that the reader will be fully aware of the clinical and diagnostic problems that they present.

FIBROCYSTIC DISEASE AND RELATED CONDITIONS

This category includes the large group of closely related lesions characterized by stromal fibrous tissue overgrowth, cystic dilatation of ducts, cyst formation, apocrine metaplasia and hyperplasia of the mammary ducts and lobules. There is great variation of opinion in the literature concerning the confines of this group of abnormalities, but in this volume they are considered together for purposes of organization and correlation with mammographic findings. Synonyms and related terms are: cystic disease, chronic cystic mastitis, mazoplasia, mammary dysplasia, Schimmelbusch's disease, adenocystic disease, fibrous mastitis and chronic mastitis.

The lesions are thought to result from exaggeration and distortion of the cyclic changes that normally occur in the breast during the menstrual cycle. They may be diffuse or localized, unilateral or bilateral. Depending on which of the morphologic components is dominant, the group can be subdivided according to five general types of lesions: (1) predominantly cystic, (2) predominantly fibrous, (3) predominantly lobular hyperplasia (adenosis), (4) predominantly ductal (intraductal epithelial hyperplasia, papillomatosis), and (5) mixed or no dominant type.

FIBROCYSTIC DISEASE—PREDOMINANTLY CYSTIC.—Fibrocystic disease of the predominately cystic type (Figs. **21–23**) is the commonest form of fibrocystic disease encountered by the surgeon. It is most frequent near or at the menopause, affecting patients 45–55 years old, but it is found in patients of all ages after sexual maturity. The lesion is characterized by dilatation of ducts and the formation of cysts, accompanied by various degrees of stromal and epithelial hyperplasia. It can occur as an isolated cyst (Fig. **24**) but usually is multifocal and often bilateral (Figs. **25–30**).

FIBROCYSTIC DISEASE—PREDOMINANTLY FIBROUS.—The predominantly fibrous type of fibrocystic disease is found with a relatively high frequency in women with diffusely nodular breasts who complain of persistent or recurring pain and soreness. It is prevalent between the ages of 30 and 50 but occurs in both younger and older patients.

The principal pathologic characteristic of this condition is a stromal fibrous tissue overgrowth often not associated with ductal hyperplasia or grossly demonstrable cysts, though both may be present. This lesion is more frequently bilateral and diffuse (Figs. **31–33**) than unilateral and isolated, but it can occur as an apparently localized lesion (Figs. **34** and **35**) in otherwise normal breasts.

The radiographic features are nonspecific and variable. For the most part, when it is bilateral, this condition is difficult to distinguish from normal breast parenchyma. The breasts tend to be somewhat more radiopaque than would be expected for the age of the patient, however, and in a minority of cases the fibrosis is so extreme that a homogeneous ground-glass appearance is present even in the breasts of postmenopausal patients. The localized variety, when seen in an otherwise fatty type of breast, frequently mimics carcinoma in radiographic appearance (Fig. **35, B–D**).

LOBULAR HYPERPLASIA (ADENOSIS, SCLEROSING ADENOSIS).—Mammary disease in which lobular hyperplasia predominates is encountered less frequently than are the cystic and fibrotic varieties. Two phases of the process are recognized. In the earlier or florid phase, lobular hyperplasia predominates (Fig. **36**), with proliferation and multiplication of ducts and formation of narrowed tubules or solid cords of cells. In the later stage, which is usually known as sclerosing adenosis (Figs. **37–39**), fibrous tissue proliferation and dense deposits of collagen surround and compress glandular lumens, resulting in formation of narrowed tubules or solid cords of cells. The lesion mimics carcinoma on both gross and microscopic examination in many cases. Focal areas of this process are often seen in advanced mixed forms of fibrocystic disease.

Adenosis is often a localized process but may be generalized. It presents as a discrete palpable mass, and it more commonly affects women between 20 and 35 years of age than it does older women. It is difficult to recognize the lesion, especially when it is in the florid phase, on mammograms of young women, as the appearance is almost indistinguishable from that of confluent deposits of normal breast parenchyma. However, in older patients and especially in patients past the menopause, it often presents as an irregular dominant mass containing flecks of calcium. In these cases it is indistinguishable from some atypical forms of carcinoma (Fig. **39**).

INTRADUCTAL EPITHELIAL HYPERPLASIA AND PAPILLOMATOSIS.—Intraductal hyperplasia and ductal papillomatosis are commonly encountered with other forms of fibrocystic disease, but occasionally they occur in isolated or predominant forms. These lesions often involve extensive areas of the small mammary ducts, especially at the lobular level. They consist of hyperplasia and papillary proliferations of the ductal epithelium. Atypical ductal hyperplasia may be a premalignant phase.

Usually, the presence of epithelial hyperplasia or papillomatosis is unsuspected on the basis of the mammogram, but in an occasional case, calcifications in the papillary lesions give a radiographic clue to their presence (Figs. **40** and **41**).

FIBROADENOMA AND CYSTOSARCOMA PHYLLOIDES

Fibroadenoma (Figs. **42–45**) is the commonest benign tumor of the breast in the age group between 20 and 35 and one of the commonest at all ages. It may develop at any age but usually manifests itself early in the child-bearing period. Fibroadenoma tends to be localized and solitary, though multiple tumors occur in about 15% of cases and diffuse forms are seen in rare instances. About 3% calcify after the menopause.

Radiographically, in a fatty type of breast a fibroadenoma presents the classic picture of a benign tumor (Fig. **42**). It is rounded or lobular, smooth walled and homogeneous. In the breasts of older patients, typical coarse calcifications are sometimes seen (Fig. **45**). In those of younger patients, in whom it is most common, the tumor is often surrounded and obscured by normal breast tissue of the same radiographic density (Fig. **43**).

Cystosarcoma phylloides, or giant fibroadenoma as it is sometimes called, is a variant of fibroadenoma which is characterized by its large size (Figs. **46** and **47**). Most behave as benign lesions, but others may be locally invasive and infiltrate the underlying muscle and chest wall. A malignant variant is found in 10% or less of the cases (Fig. **47, B**). This lesion shows all the histologic changes of a fibrosarcoma.

There are no specific radiographic criteria except size that differentiate fibroadenoma from cystosarcoma phylloides. The malignant variant may show evidence of invasion of surrounding tissues in some cases.

INTRADUCTAL PAPILLOMA

Among the benign tumors affecting the breast, benign intraductal papilloma (Fig. **48**) is one of the lesions most frequently encountered in clinical practice. In many instances, these lesions are accompanied by serous or sanguineous discharge from the nipple. They occur at any age but are seen only rarely before 20 and after 65. Multiple lesions are common. They are usually small, seldom exceeding 1–2 cm in diameter. Rarely, large lesions are encountered (Fig. **49**). They can be located anywhere in the ductal system, but most are found in the larger lactiferous ducts beneath the nipple.

Most intraductal papillomas are not visible as discrete masses on the mammogram. In my experience, most of them cannot be identified, as they are obscured by dense subareolar tissues. In fatty breasts, however, their location often can be determined by the dilatation of the lactiferous ducts which harbor them (Fig. **48, A**). In unusual instances they are visible as small discrete masses which may contain calcifications (Fig. **48, B** and **C**).

MISCELLANEOUS BENIGN TUMORS AND TUMOR-LIKE LESIONS

GYNECOMASTIA.—Enlargement of the male breast (gynecomastia) results from proliferation and hyperplasia of both stromal and parenchymal tissues of the breast in response to excesses of estrogen. This abnormality is often seen as a side-effect of stilbestrol therapy for carcinoma of the prostate gland and whenever there is a cause for hyperestrinism. It frequently occurs in otherwise normal individuals at puberty and in very old age. There is no relationship between carcinoma and gynecomastia.

Two types are recognized on the mammograms. One consists of fatty enlargement of the breast with no radiographic evidence of stromal or parenchymal growth. The second and more common type (Fig. **50**) consists of a proliferation of glandular tissue beneath the nipple which produces a nodular mass suggesting fibrocystic disease. This lesion is not ordinarily confused with carcinoma because of its regular margins and homogeneous density, but in some instances it is irregular in outline, mimicking carcinoma in appearance.

PLASMA CELL MASTITIS.—This rare granulomatous type of process is obscure in origin but is thought by many to be primarily chemical rather than bacterial in nature and to result from stasis and inspissation of secretions. It occurs most frequently in multiparous women who give a history of difficult nursing. There is no clear-cut distinction between this disease and mammary duct ectasia (comedomastitis). Clinically and histologically, plasma cell mastitis is difficult to distinguish from carcinoma: in some instances, it produces an irregular density beneath the nipple, which mimics carcinoma; also, nipple retraction and skin thickening may be present. In other cases (Fig. **51**), a more circumscribed lesion is seen.

MAMMARY DUCT ECTASIA (COMEDOMASTITIS).—Mammary duct ectasia is characterized pathologically by dilatation of ducts, inspissation of ductal secretions, periductal inflammation and stromal fibrosis. As was just mentioned, this condition is not clearly distinguished from plasma cell mastitis in some cases, but in its advanced stages it produces a characteristic radiographic appearance (Fig. **52**). The mammogram in most instances shows a dense subareolar fibrosis, often accompanied by nipple retraction. Calcifications are usually present and are distinctive. These consist of coarse linear and ringlike deposits which occur in the walls of the ducts deep to the nipple, but in some cases may be seen distributed widely throughout the glandular portions of the breast.

GALACTOCELE.—Galactocele is a cystic dilatation of a mammary duct which develops during lactation, probably as the result of ductal obstruction. The cysts may be solitary (Fig. **53**), multiple or multiloculated. Early in their development they contain a colostrum-like material and have thin smooth walls. Later, a thick cheese-like material is found, and the wall may be thickened due to inflammation. On the mammogram, the galactocele is radiolucent, because of its content of fatty colostrum-like material, and stands out in sharp contrast to the surrounding radiopaque lactating breast tissue. At times, the lesion persists after lactation.

LIPOMA.—Nodular accumulations of fat and true lipomas are common in large fatty breasts. Clinically, they often present as dominant masses. In most instances, they cannot be identified as discrete lesions on the mammogram, but in some cases, they have a fibrous capsule which is visible on the radiograph (Fig. 54).

HEMATOMA.—Hematoma of the breast is seen most frequently after excisional biopsy, but occasionally it results from external trauma. The collection of blood usually appears on the mammogram as an irregular opaque mass (Fig. 55) which mimics carcinoma.

BREAST PROSTHESIS AND AUGMENTATION MAMMOPLASTY.—Augmentation mammoplasty produces various roentgenographic appearances, according to the technique used. Whereas an Ivalon-sponge prosthesis appears clearly demarcated (Fig. 56, A), augmentation of breast size by liquid silicone produces (1) a nodular pattern of increased density with ovoid masses throughout the breast or (2) a more homogeneous density with no discrete masses.[1]

Techniques involving the use of autologous tissue are more likely to have various natural appearances—cystic, fibrotic and calcific (Fig. 56, B).

BENIGN TUMORS AND TUMOR-LIKE LESIONS OF THE SKIN.—A wide variety of benign tumors of the skin are seen on the mammogram (Fig. 57). In most instances, radiographic diagnosis is not difficult, but if the radiologist is unaware of the presence of a lesion on the skin, he easily may confuse it with an intramammary tumor.

INFLAMMATORY DISEASE

Inflammatory diseases of the breast are, on the whole, relatively uncommon. They are most prevalent in lactating women but are observed at any age. Acute bacterial infections and nonspecific acute mastitis of undetermined etiology are seen with greatest frequency, but virtually any type of inflammatory process can occur.

Most inflammatory lesions, especially when they are acute and of bacterial origin, can be distinguished from carcinoma on the basis of a history of acute onset with pain, tenderness and fever, but others present a less characteristic clinical picture and frequently mimic carcinoma.

On the mammogram, inflammatory lesions are usually characterized by

---

[1] Minagi, H.; Youker, J. E., and Knudson, H. W.: Radiology 90:57, 1968.

thickening of the skin, disruption of the architectural pattern of the parenchyma, increased vascularity of the breast and often by the presence of an irregular or ill-defined mass (Figs. **58–62**). These characteristics are identical with the radiographic characteristics of carcinoma and more specifically of carcinoma in its diffuse or inflammatory forms. In my experience, most acute inflammatory lesions have been incorrectly diagnosed as carcinoma because of this similarity.

Figure 21.—Fibrocystic disease—localized cysts.

A palpable mass in the left breast of a 53-year-old woman proved on biopsy to be fibrocystic disease with multiple cysts.

Two cysts (**a**) with very little surrounding stromal fibrosis are visible in the central portion of the breast. The remainder of the breast is of the fatty type. Prominent lactiferous ducts (**b**) are seen deep to the nipple.

These lesions present the classic radiographic characteristics of benign cysts: (1) The margins are clearly defined and smooth. (2) The mass is homogeneously dense throughout. (3) A thin radiolucent line representing a halo of fat surrounds the mass. (4) More than one lesion is present.

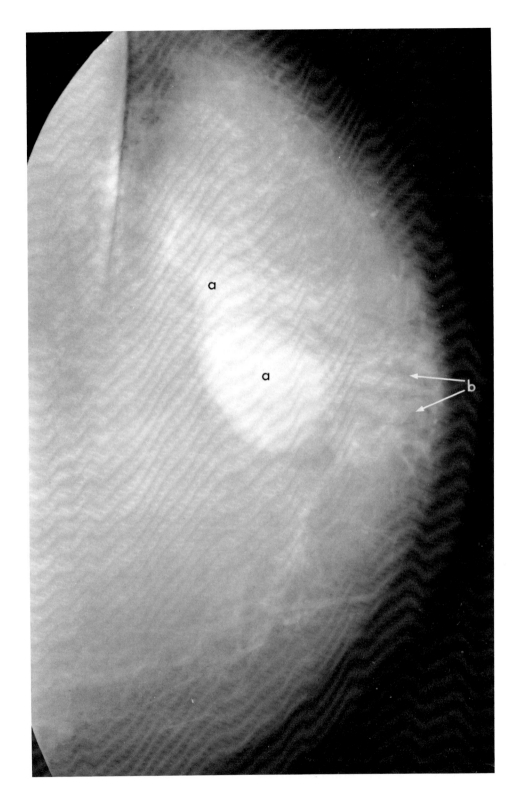

Figure 21 · Localized Cysts / 55

Figure 22.—Fibrocystic disease—localized cysts with surrounding fibrosis.

A 50-year-old woman had a mass in the right breast known to be present for 2 months. Several small cysts, the largest of which measured 1.5 cm in diameter, were found at operation.

Stromal fibrosis of varying severity accompanies cyst formation in almost every case. In this example, the surrounding fibrotic tissue (**arrows**) partially obscures the margins of the underlying cysts.

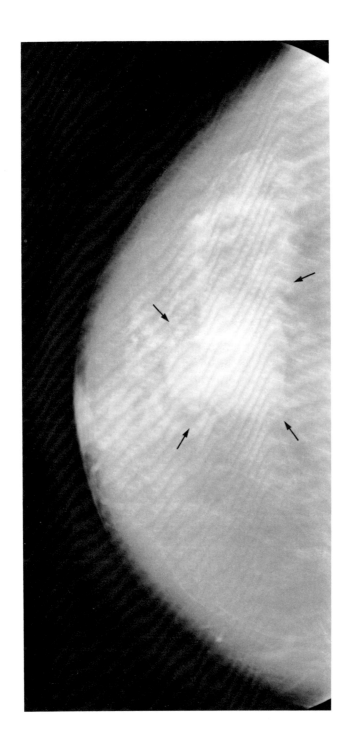

Figure 23.—Fibrocystic disease—localized subareolar cyst with dense surrounding fibrosis.

A 54-year-old woman had a tender mass in the right breast beneath the edge of the areola. Clinically a cyst, the lesion was aspirated and air injected into it.

A, mediolateral view before aspiration: Because of a dense area of fibrosis (**arrows**) beneath the areola and nipple, the underlying cyst cannot be identified on the mammogram.

B, craniocaudal view after aspiration and injection of air: The small smooth-walled cyst (**arrow**) is well demonstrated against its background of fibrous tissue.

Figure 23, courtesy of Dr. G. M. Stevens, Palo Alto Clinic, Palo Alto, Calif.

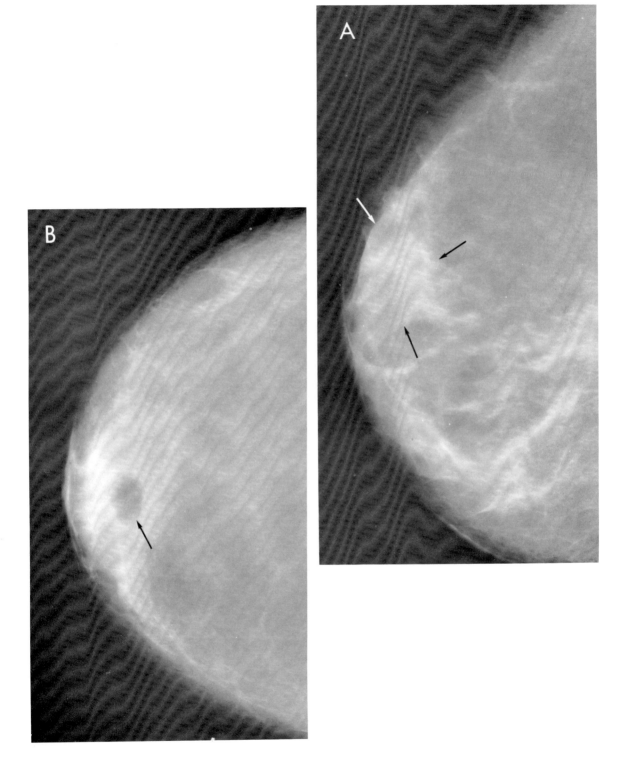

Figure 23 · Subareolar Cyst with Fibrosis / 59

Figure 24.—Fibrocystic disease—large solitary cyst with surrounding fibrosis.

A 49-year-old woman had a large mass in the upper portion of the left breast. A cyst had been removed previously from the right breast. At operation, a large cyst measuring 6 × 5 cm was found associated with extensive fibrosis and several small cysts about 0.5 cm in diameter.

A, craniocaudal view: The large cyst (**arrows**) is demonstrated, but not the smaller cysts, and the margins of the mass are obscured by surrounding dense fibrous tissue. Due to the indistinct character of the cyst wall, well-circumscribed carcinoma cannot be excluded.

B, mediolateral view: The anterior margin of the cyst (**arrows**) is clearly defined and smooth, suggesting the benign nature of the lesion.

This case illustrates the importance of viewing a mass in more than one projection to determine its radiographic characteristics.

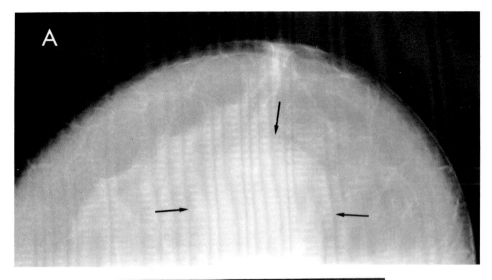

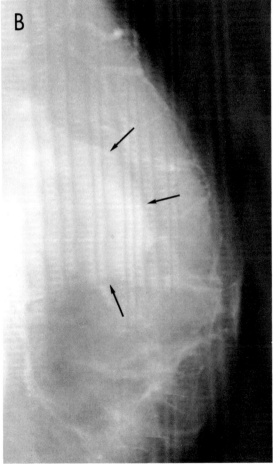

Figure 24 · Large Cyst with Fibrosis / 61

Figure 25.—Fibrocystic disease—multiple cysts scattered throughout the breast.

Multiple palpable masses in the left breast of a 49-year-old woman were clinically benign. At operation, multiple cysts up to 3 cm in diameter were excised.

The mammogram of this typical diffuse type of fibrocystic disease shows a few scattered cysts (**arrows**) throughout the breast. Relatively little associated stromal fibrosis is seen.

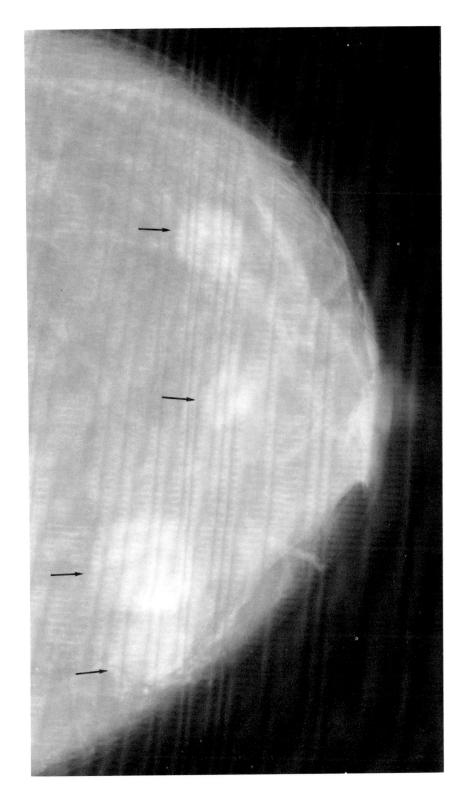

Figure 25 · Multiple Cysts Throughout / 63

Figure 26.—Fibrocystic disease of diffuse type with multiple cysts.

Multiple masses in the right breast of a 49-year-old woman seemed to represent fibrocystic disease clinically. The lesions were aspirated and air was injected.

A, mammogram before aspiration: Diffuse fibrocystic disease involves the entire breast, with multiple cysts (**arrows**) in the upper part of the breast. Much overlapping of the cysts is present, but where seen, the margins appear to be typically benign.

B, mammogram after aspiration and injection of air: At least two cysts were not aspirated. The walls of the air-filled cysts (**arrows**) are thin and smooth. Note that the outlines of the cysts tend to be somewhat lobulated or ovoid, not smoothly rounded.

Figure 26, courtesy of Dr. G. M. Stevens, Palo Alto Clinic, Palo Alto, Calif.

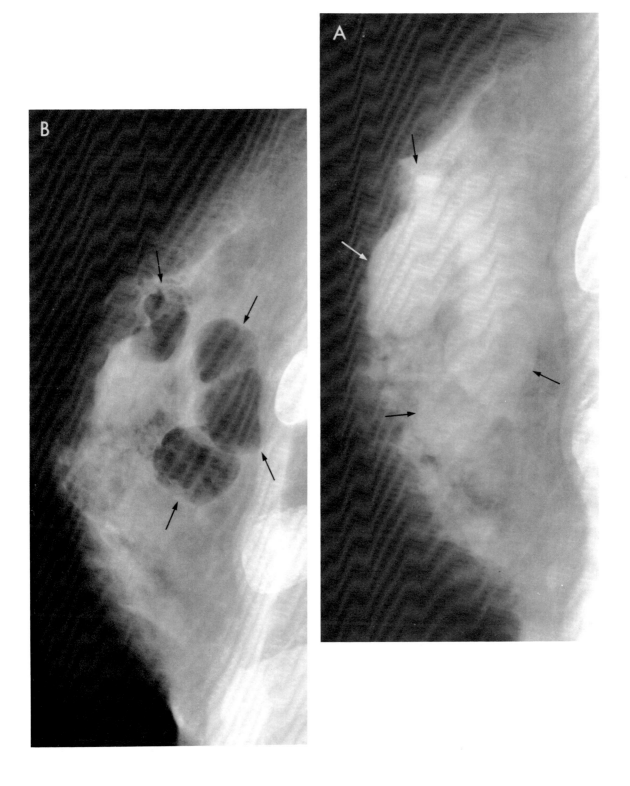

Figure 26 · Diffuse Fibrocystic Disease / 65

Figure 27.—Fibrocystic disease of diffuse type with small cysts and scattered calcifications.

A discrete mass was palpable in the upper outer portion of the right breast of a 45-year-old woman with a long history of bilateral diffuse fibrocystic disease. Biopsy showed fibrocystic disease with multiple small cysts, stromal fibrosis and some areas of hyperplasia of the ductal epithelium.

A, entire breast, craniocaudal view: Diffuse fibrocystic disease of moderate degree is evident. Scattered punctate calcifications (**a**) are present throughout much of the breast.

B, enlarged segment of mammogram: The punctate calcifications (**a**) are typical of many cases of fibrocystic disease. The calcifications are rounded, scattered in a random fashion throughout the breast and of relatively uniform size. Care must be taken to distinguish this type of calcification from the calcification of carcinoma (see Chap. 4).

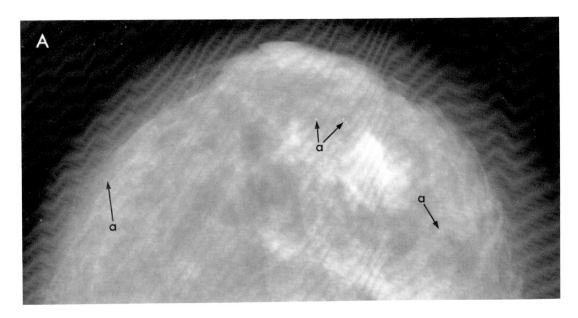

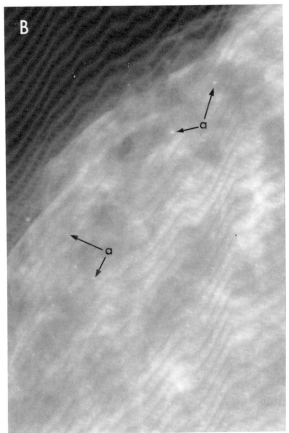

Figure 27 · Diffuse Fibrocystic Disease, Calcifications / 67

Figure 28—Fibrocystic disease—diffuse, combined cystic and fibrotic type.

Both breasts of a 22-year-old woman contained multiple masses. Biopsy showed a mixed type of fibrocystic disease with prominent cysts up to 1 cm in diameter, extensive stromal fibrosis and some regions of adenosis.

A, mediolateral view.

B, craniocaudal view.

The breast is radiopaque and has a ground-glass appearance. Cysts cannot be identified. The appearance is quite similar to that of the normal breast during the early reproductive years (see Fig. 12, p. 29).

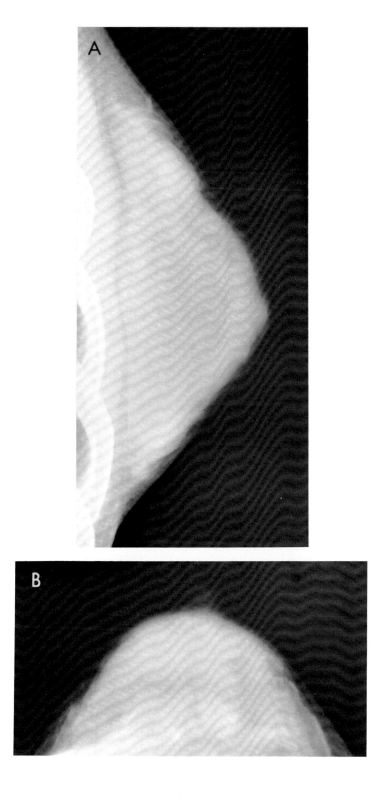

Figure 28 · Diffuse Fibrocystic Disease / 69

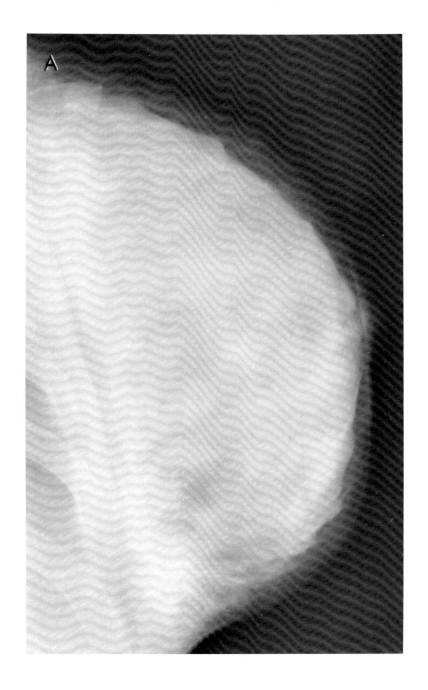

70 / **Figure 29** · **Diffuse Fibrocystic Disease, Premenopausal**

Figure 29.—Fibrocystic disease—diffuse, predominantly cystic type.

A 37-year-old woman complained of pain in the breasts. Both breasts were nodular throughout on physical examination. Biopsy showed multiple cysts, varying from 0.4 to 1 cm in diameter, and regions of dense stromal fibrosis and adenosis.

A, mediolateral view.

B, craniocaudal view.

The breast is dense and nodular throughout. Individual cysts cannot be identified with certainty, and no dominant mass is seen.

This case illustrates the typical radiographic appearance of the most common type of fibrocystic disease seen in the premenopausal woman. The breasts of these women are difficult to evaluate by mammography, and because of the presence of extensive benign disease, carcinoma when present is often obscured.

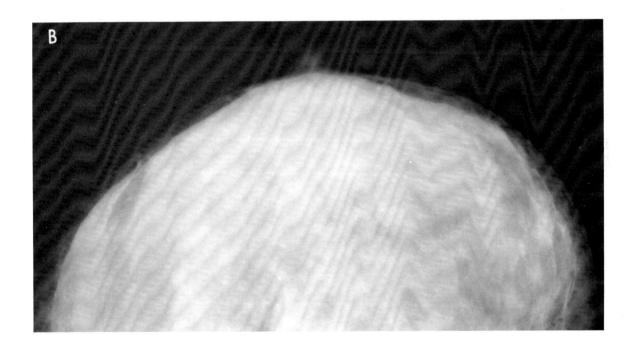

Figure 29 · Diffuse Fibrocystic Disease, Premenopausal / 71

Figure 30.—Fibrocystic disease in a postmenopausal patient.

A mass in the left breast was noted on routine physical examination of a 62-year-old woman, 10 years after the menopause. Biopsy showed a localized area of fibrocystic disease measuring $8 \times 4.5 \times 4.5$ cm. Several cysts ranging up to 1.5 cm in diameter were present.

The mammogram shows a lobular, circumscribed mass (**arrows**). The appearance is that of a benign process, but no distinctive radiographic characteristics which would identify the type of lesion are seen.

Fibrocystic disease rarely if ever develops after the menopause. However, lesions which develop before the menopause frequently persist in the postmenopausal patient. I have observed diffuse fibrocystic disease, proved by biopsy, in the breast of a 90-year-old woman.

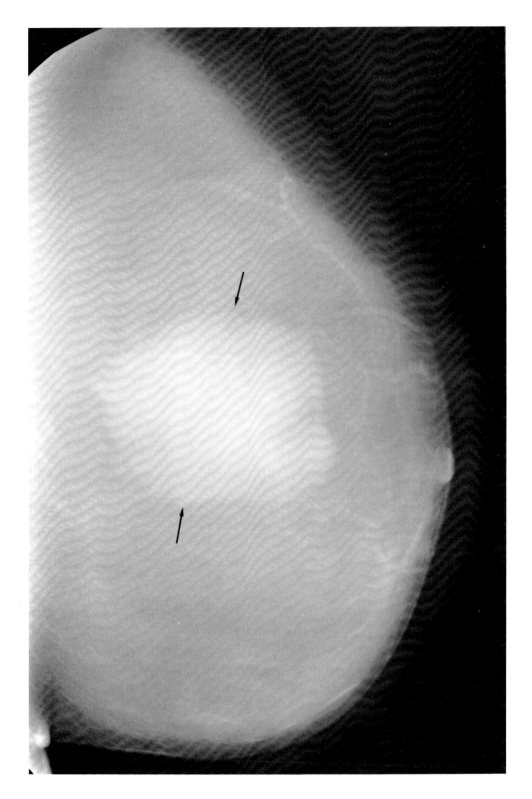

Figure 30 · Fibrocystic Disease, Postmenopausal / 73

Figure 31.—Fibrocystic disease—diffuse, predominantly fibrous type.

The breasts of a 36-year-old patient with mastodynia were firm to palpation and diffusely nodular. At biopsy, the diffuse, fibrous type of fibrocystic disease was found.

The radiographic density of the breast tissue is greater than would ordinarily be expected in a patient of this age. There is a tendency to a homogeneous ground-glass appearance, although several areas of prominent nodular parenchyma are seen.

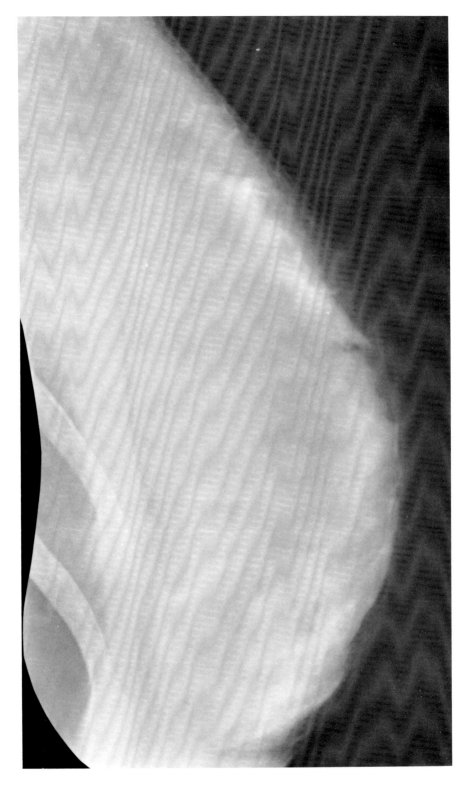

Figure 31 · Diffuse Fibrous Type Fibrocystic Disease / 75

Figure 32.—Fibrocystic disease—diffuse, predominantly fibrous type.

A 45-year-old woman had painful and tender breasts. On palpation no dominant mass was evident, but the breasts were hard and finely nodular throughout. Biopsy showed diffuse dense fibrosis and multiple tiny cysts less than 5 mm in diameter.

A, mediolateral view.

B, craniocaudal view.

The breasts have an opaque ground-glass appearance. Subcutaneous fat is sparse. Several deposits of both coarse and fine calcification (**arrows**) are present. The appearance mimics that seen in the adolescent breast.

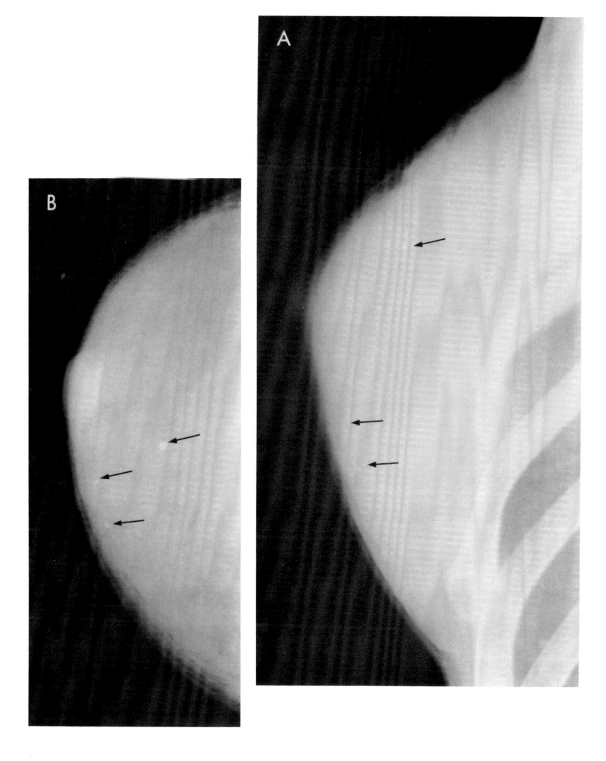

Figure 32 · Diffuse Fibrous Type Fibrocystic Disease / 77

Figure 33.—Fibrocystic disease—diffuse, predominantly fibrous type.

A mass in the tail of the breast of a 44-year-old woman was suspected clinically to be carcinoma. Biopsy showed fibrocystic disease of the predominantly fibrous type with ductal calcification.

Craniocaudal view: The breast parenchyma has the homogeneous appearance commonly seen in this condition. An extensive area of calcification (**arrows**) is present in the lateral half of the breast. Most of the calcifications are coarse and rounded, suggesting benign disease.

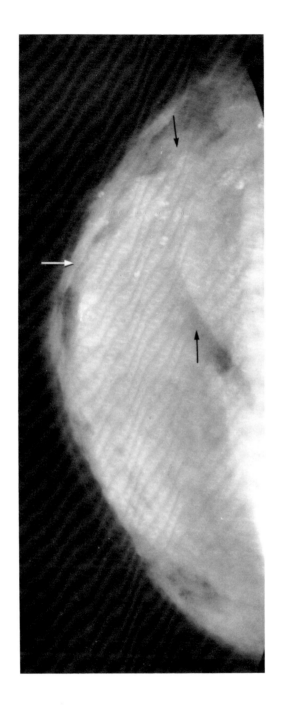

Figure 33 · Diffuse Fibrous Type Fibrocystic Disease / 79

Figure 34.—Fibrocystic disease—localized, predominantly fibrous type.

A 63-year-old woman had had previous mastectomy on the right for carcinoma. A mass was palpable in the upper outer portion of the left breast. Biopsy showed localized fibrocystic disease, predominantly of the fibrous type but with associated focal areas of sclerosing adenosis, intraductal papillomatosis, intraductal epithelial hyperplasia and apocrine metaplasia.

Nodular fibrous-appearing parenchyma presents as a dominant mass on the mammogram. Most of the rest of the breast is of the atrophic, fatty type. A few rounded punctate calcifications (**a**) are seen within the area of fibrosis (**arrows**).

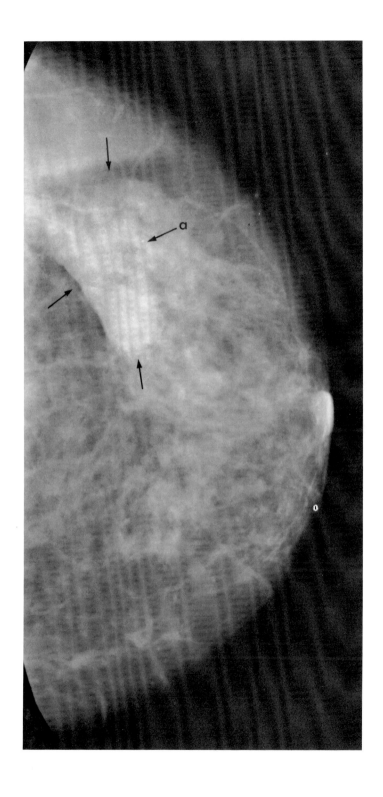

Figure 34 · Localized Fibrous Fibrocystic Disease / 81

Figure 35.—Fibrocystic disease—localized, predominantly fibrous type presenting as dominant mass.

A palpable mass in the right breast of a 67-year-old woman, proved on biopsy to be localized fibrocystic disease of the fibrous type. No gross cysts were present.

A, on the mammogram, the lesion mimics fibroadenoma.

A palpable mass in the left breast of a 72-year-old woman was suspected clinically to be carcinoma. Simple mastectomy was performed, but only localized fibrous type of fibrocystic disease was found.

B, the lesion (**arrows**) is irregular and presents as a stellate mass containing a single coarse calcification. It cannot be distinguished from carcinoma.

The remaining breast of a 43-year-old woman who had had previous mastectomy for carcinoma was asymptomatic. Simple mastectomy was performed on the basis of the mammogram. Only localized fibrocystic disease was found.

C, the lesion (**arrows**) on the mammogram mimics a small infiltrating carcinoma.

A 65-year-old woman had a clinically indeterminate mass in the breast. Biopsy showed localized fibrocystic disease of the fibrous type.

D, radiographically, the lesion (**arrows**) mimics carcinoma of the scirrhous type and cannot be differentiated from it.

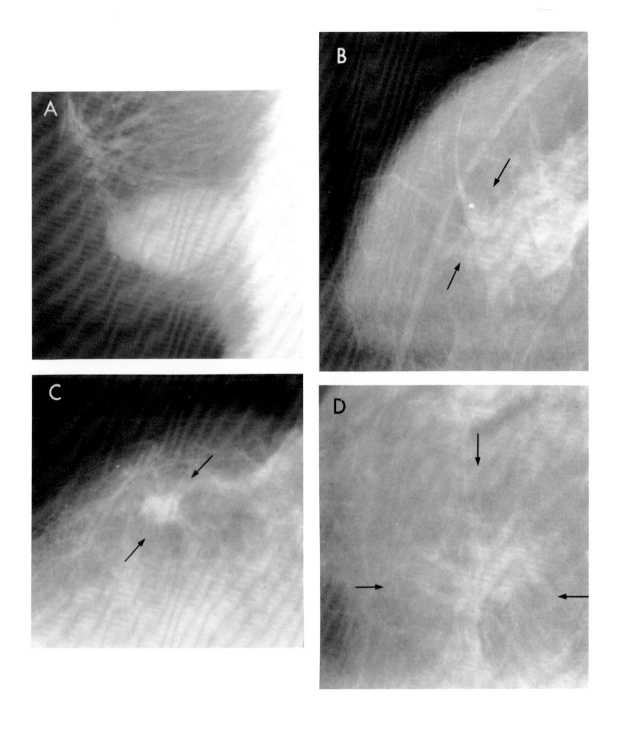

Figure 35 · Localized Fibrous Fibrocystic Disease / 83

Figure 36.—Lobular hyperplasia (adenosis).

A firm 4 cm nodular mass in the upper outer quadrant of the left breast of a 30-year-old woman had been present for at least 6 weeks. Biopsy disclosed adenosis of the florid type.

On the mammogram, an ill-defined area of increased density with no discrete margins represents the region of the palpable mass (**a**). Other smaller though similar deposits are present in the middle (**b**) and lower (**c**) parts of the breast. It is not possible to differentiate between normal breast tissue and adenosis in this case.

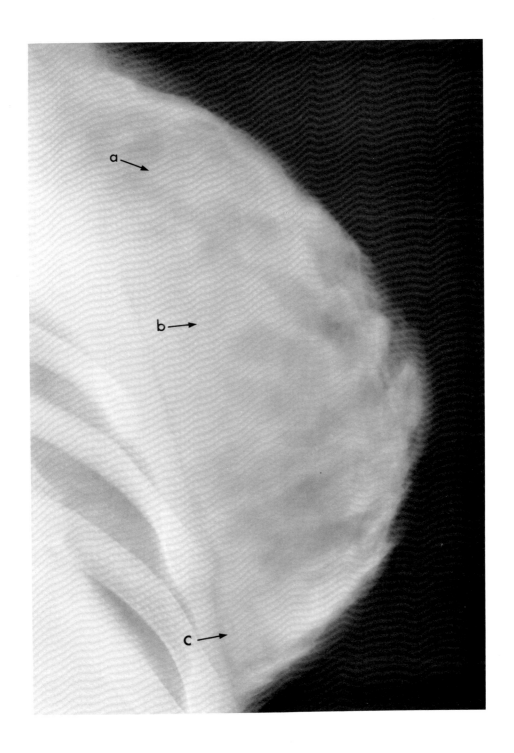

Figure 36 · Lobular Hyperplasia (Adenosis) / 85

Figure 37.—Fibrocystic disease—diffuse mixed type with multiple foci of sclerosing adenosis.

A 67-year-old woman had diffusely nodular breasts, but a more discrete palpable nodule was present in the 12 o'clock position on the right. Biopsy demonstrated diffuse fibrocystic disease with focal deposits of sclerosing adenosis.

The right breast presents a diffusely nodular pattern, and an area of irregular increased density in the 12 o'clock position (**arrow**). A few tiny flecks of calcium could be identified in this area on the original film.

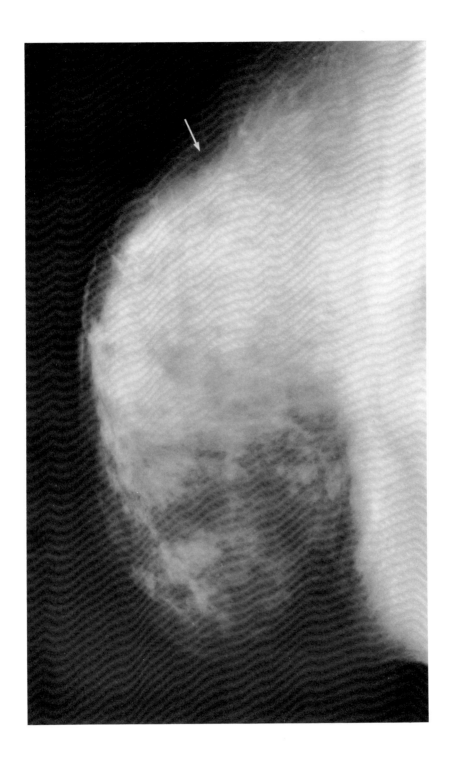

Figure 37 · Fibrocystic Disease, Sclerosing Adenosis / 87

Figure 38.—Sclerosing adenosis—localized type, mimicking carcinoma.

A mass in the left breast of a 61-year-old woman had clinical characteristics suggesting carcinoma. Biopsy showed sclerosing adenosis associated with intraductal hyperplasia in a region of fibrocystic disease of the fibrous type.

A, entire breast, craniocaudal view.

B, localized segment of the lesion, mediolateral projection.

The mass (**arrow**) is irregular in outline with a tendency to spiculation. In **B,** prominent veins (**a**) are seen in the region of the mass. The appearance mimics that of circumscribed carcinoma.

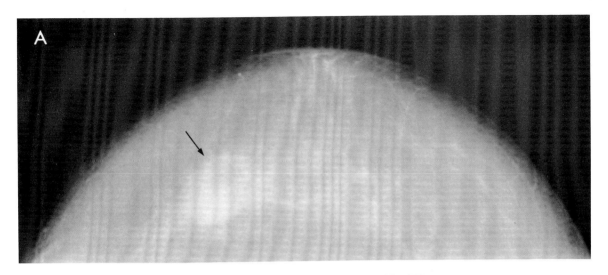

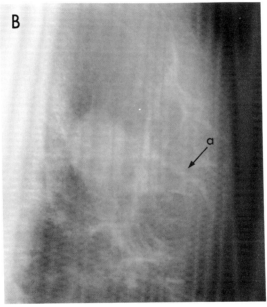

Figure 38 · Localized Sclerosing Adenosis / 89

Figure 39.—Sclerosing adenosis—localized type, mimicking carcinoma.

A hard movable mass was palpable in the right breast of a 47-year-old woman. Biopsy showed one large and several smaller areas of sclerosing adenosis with associated intraductal hyperplasia and calcification.

A, entire breast, mediolateral view.

B, localized enlarged segment, craniocaudal view.

Irregular, punctate calcifications (**arrows**) of varying size are seen in and around the mass in the upper part of the breast. The margins of the mass are somewhat irregular, suggesting well-circumscribed carcinoma. The calcifications are indistinguishable from those seen in carcinoma.

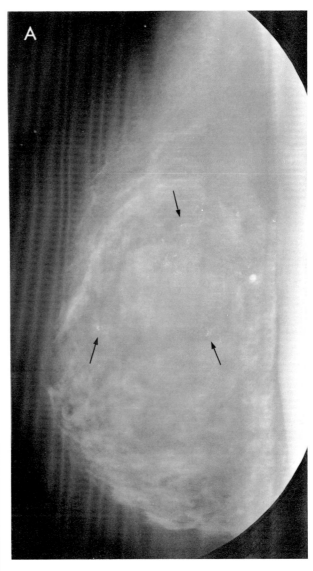

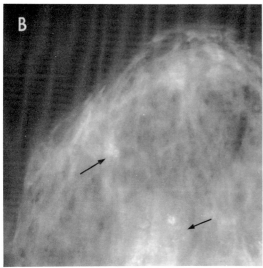

Figure 39 · Localized Sclerosing Adenosis / 91

Figure 40.—Fibrocystic disease—diffuse fibrous type with ductal hyperplasia.

On physical examination, a nodule was detected in the upper part of the left breast of a 49-year-old woman with mastodynia. Biopsy showed diffuse fibrocystic disease of the predominantly fibrous type with foci of sclerosing adenosis, intraductal hyperplasia and intraductal calcification.

Craniocaudal view: The breast is diffusely radiopaque, giving a picture compatible with diffuse fibrocystic disease of the fibrous type. Punctate calcifications are seen (**a**), giving the only clue to the presence of intraductal epithelial hyperplasia.

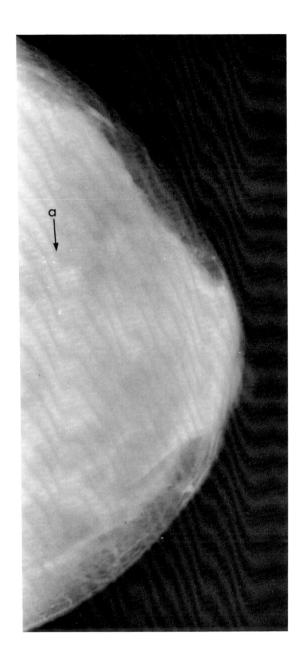

Figure 40 · Intraductal Epithelial Hyperplasia / 93

Figure 41.—Ductal papillomatosis.

No lesion was palpable on physical examination of a 63-year-old asymptomatic woman. Biopsy, performed on the basis of the mammographic suggestion of possible intraductal carcinoma, showed fibrocystic disease with proliferative changes including papillomatosis and adenosis. Epithelial and intraductal calcifications were present.

A, entire breast, craniocaudal view.

B, enlarged section of mammogram to show detail of calcifications.

Calcifications of various sizes (**arrows**) are the only evidence of extensive intraductal papillomatosis. Many of these calcifications appear rounded and suggest benign disease, but the variation in size and the irregular appearance of many of the calcific flecks make it difficult to distinguish this lesion from carcinoma.

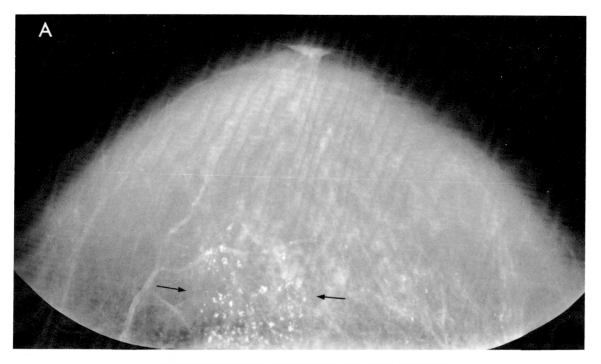

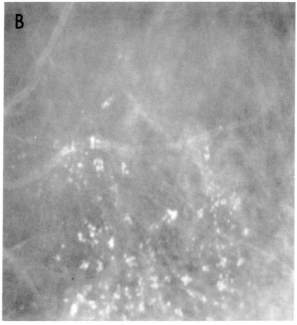

Figure 41 · Ductal Papillomatosis / 95

Figure 42.—Fibroadenoma.

Biopsy of the left breast of a 73-year-old asymptomatic woman with multiple masses in both breasts revealed multiple calcified and uncalcified fibroadenomas.

This mammogram depicts the classic radiographic features of fibro-adenoma. The lesions are rounded but tend toward lobulation. The wall is otherwise smooth and regular. The tumors are homogeneously radiopaque throughout, and typical coarse dense calcification is present in some.

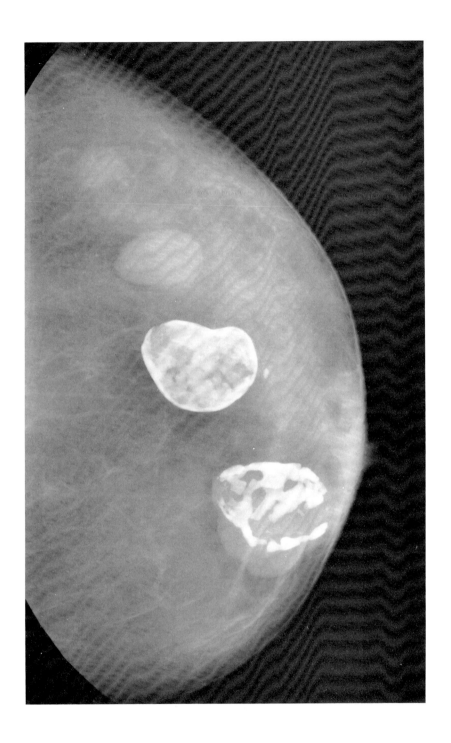

Figure 42 · Fibroadenoma / 97

Figure 43.—Fibroadenoma.

A mass in the left breast of a 20-year-old unmarried woman was firm, movable and discrete on palpation. Biopsy revealed two fibroadenomas, one measuring 2 cm in diameter, the other 1.5 cm.

A, entire breast, mediolateral view.

B, localized compression spot view of the tumor region.

The larger fibroadenoma (**a**) is partially obscured by surrounding normal breast tissue, and the smaller cannot be identified. The compression spot film (**B**) shows to better advantage the smooth wall and homogeneous density of the lesion (**arrows**).

In my experience, less than half of the fibroadenomas found in the breasts of young patients can be seen on the mammogram because of the presence of dense surrounding breast parenchyma.

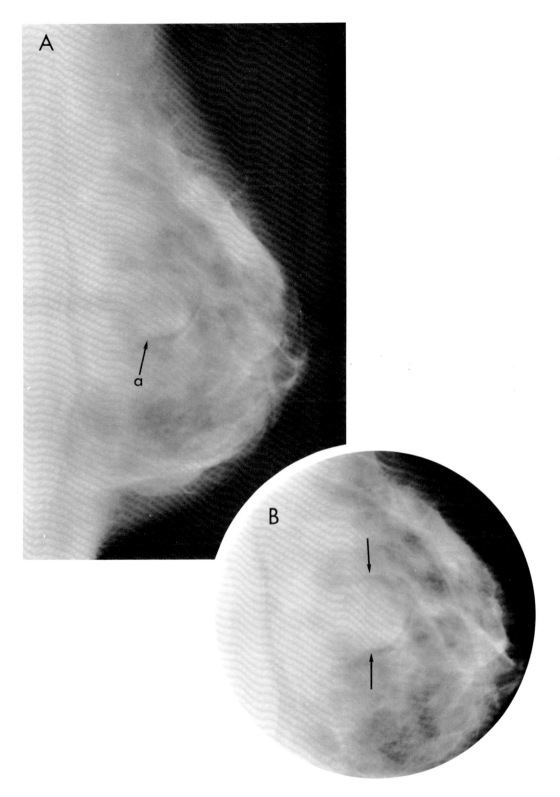

Figure 43 · Fibroadenoma / 99

Figure 44.—Fibroadenoma—variations in radiographic appearance.

A mass in the left breast of a 57-year-old woman had increased in size during a 6-month period. Biopsy showed a multicentric cellular fibroadenoma which measured 7 cm in greatest diameter.

A, craniocaudal view: The irregularity and lack of circumscription of the wall of this lesion (**arrows**) make it difficult to distinguish it from well-circumscribed carcinoma.

An asymptomatic mass in the left breast of a 44-year-old woman proved to be "early" fibroadenoma with a poorly defined capsule.

B, localized compression film: The margin of the lesion (**arrow**) fades into the surrounding breast parenchyma.

A discrete lobular mass in the medial aspect of the right breast of a 44-year-old woman proved on biopsy to be a multilobular intracanalicular fibroadenoma measuring 4 × 2 × 1.5 cm.

C, localized segment, craniocaudal view: The lesion (**arrow**) is somewhat more lobulated than most fibroadenomas, but the lobulation, circumscription and homogeneous density do suggest fibroadenoma.

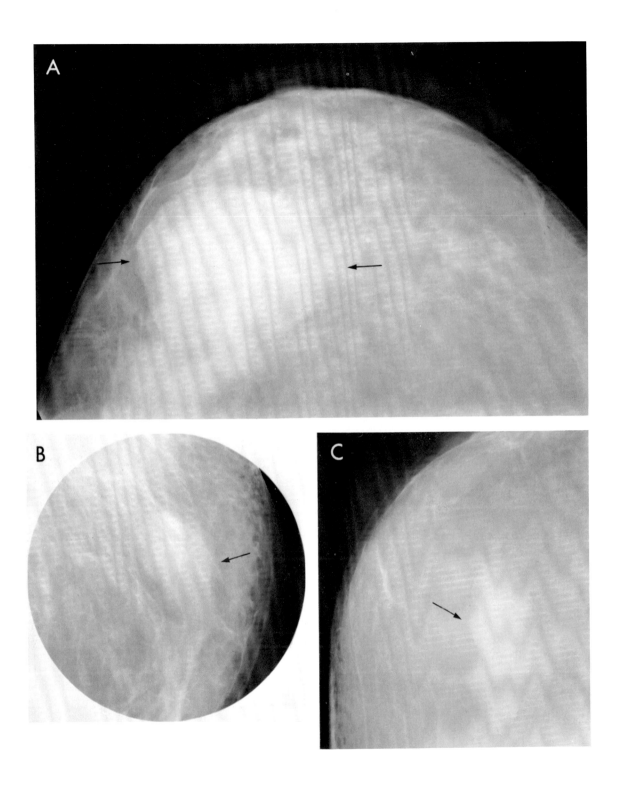

Figure 44 · Fibroadenoma: Variable Appearance / 101

Figure 45.—Fibroadenoma—variations in pattern of calcification.

A, craniocaudal view: A large fibroadenoma in the breast of a 75-year-old woman contains coarse irregular calcifications (**arrows**).

B, a small fibroadenoma in the breast of a 65-year-old woman is almost completely calcified (**a**). A small carcinoma is present beside the fibroadenoma (**b**).

C, craniocaudal view: Multiple poorly demonstrated small fibroadenomas in the breast of a 59-year-old woman contain focal calcifications (**arrows**). This lesion is difficult to differentiate from heavily calcified carcinoma.

D, a poorly circumscribed fibroadenoma in the breast of a 65-year-old woman contains coarse and irregular calcifications (**arrows**).

Figure 45, *A,* from Witten, D. M.: Minnesota Medicine 47:249, 1964; by permission of Minnesota State Medical Association.

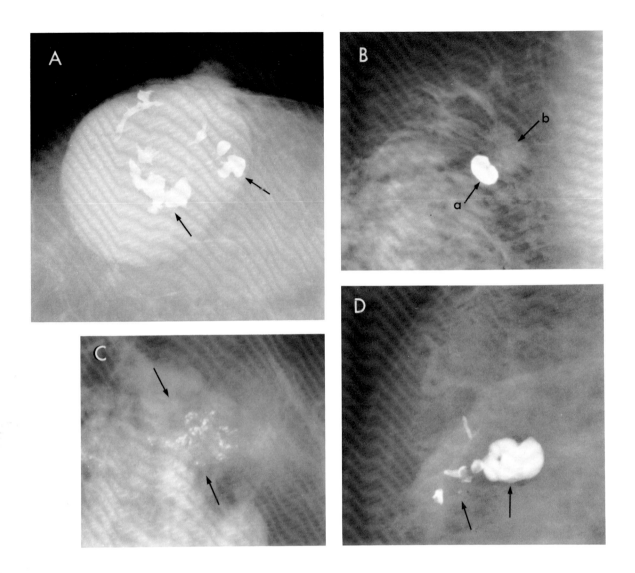

Figure 45 · Fibroadenoma, Calcifications / 103

Figure 46.—Cystosarcoma phylloides.

A large lobular mass filled the entire left breast of a 48-year-old unmarried woman. Clinically, this seemed to be a malignant lesion. Simple mastectomy was performed, and the lesion proved to be a benign lobular cystosarcoma phylloides, measuring 15 cm in greatest diameter.

Craniocaudal view: The large lobular mass is homogeneous, but its margins (**arrows**) do not appear well circumscribed. The lack of skin thickening and lack of evidence of increased vascularity of the breast are useful signs which help to differentiate this tumor from cancer.

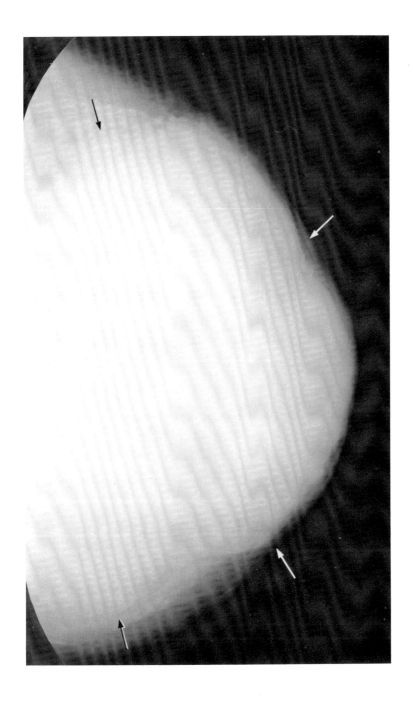

Figure 46 · Cystosarcoma Phylloides / 105

Figure 47.—Cystosarcoma phylloides.

Excisional biopsy of a large lobular mass in the left breast of a 50-year-old woman was performed. The pathologist considered the lesion to be a giant intracanalicular fibroadenoma (cystosarcoma phylloides), although it measured only 5 cm in greatest diameter.

A, the grossly lobular well-circumscribed character of the lesion (**arrows**) and the coarse calcification within it suggest fibroadenoma. The differentiation between fibroadenoma and cystosarcoma phylloides must be made by the pathologist.

An enlarging mass in the right breast of a 77-year-old woman was firm but not fixed to the chest wall. Surgery was performed, and the lesion, measuring 4 cm, proved to be a fairly well encapsulated, grade 2 malignant fibroadenoma (cystosarcoma phylloides).

B, the irregular outline of this lesion (**arrows**) suggests malignant disease, and a radiographic diagnosis of well-circumscribed carcinoma was made.

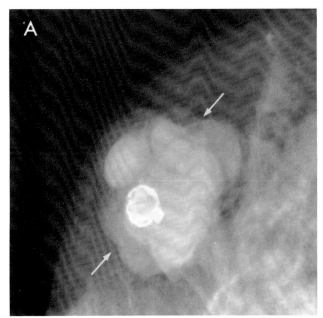

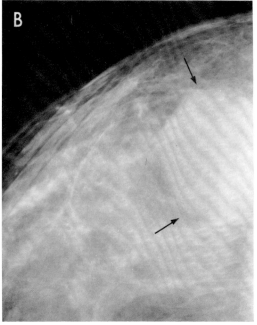

Figure 47 · Cystosarcoma Phylloides / 107

Figure 48.—Intraductal papilloma.

A benign intraductal papilloma, 1 cm in diameter, was removed from the breast of a 67-year-old woman who had a bloody discharge from one nipple.

A, craniocaudal view: The ductal thickening (**a**) seen beneath the nipple (**b**) is typical of some cases of papilloma. The lesion itself is not visible. In the presence of dense subareolar tissue, this lesion cannot be demonstrated.

A small soft mass was palpable beneath the edge of the areola of an 80-year-old woman who had a bloody discharge from one nipple. A 1 cm, cellular benign papilloma containing calcifications was found at operation.

B, craniocaudal view: Dilated subareolar lactiferous ducts (**a**) and a small mass containing flecks of calcium (**b**) are visible. The location and the presence of calcifications of the benign type suggest the diagnosis.

No mass was palpable in the breast of a 63-year-old woman who had a serosanguineous discharge from one nipple. Biopsy revealed calcified intraductal papilloma.

C, the unusually coarse calcification (**arrow**) in the tumor is the only evidence of its presence.

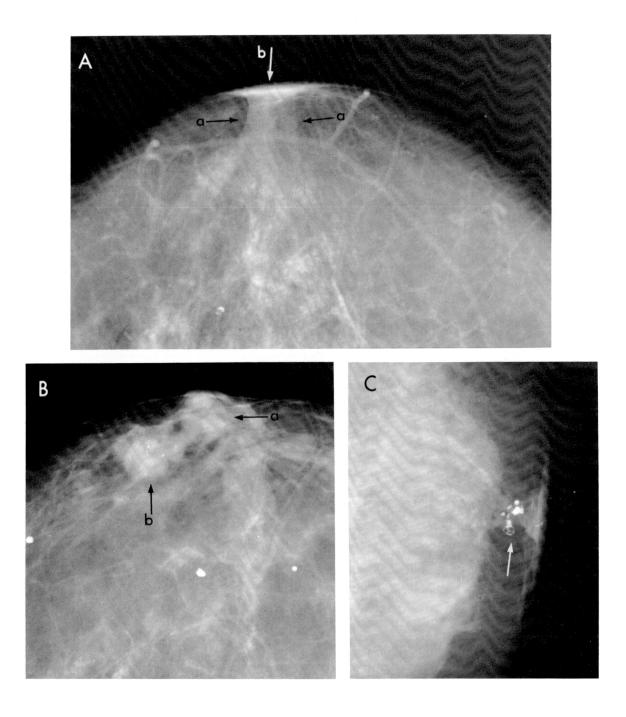

Figure 48 · Intraductal Papilloma / 109

Figure 49.—Intraductal papilloma, unusually large.

Biopsy of a palpable, 3 cm mass beneath the right nipple of a 65-year-old woman revealed a circumscribed papillary adenomatous nodule, 2.5 cm in diameter, with areas of apocrine metaplasia.

A, entire breast, craniocaudal view: A large well-circumscribed mass (**a**) is seen beneath the areola. Some nipple retraction is present (**b**).

B, enlarged segment to show the sharply marginated lesion (**arrows**). The appearance suggests cyst or fibroadenoma.

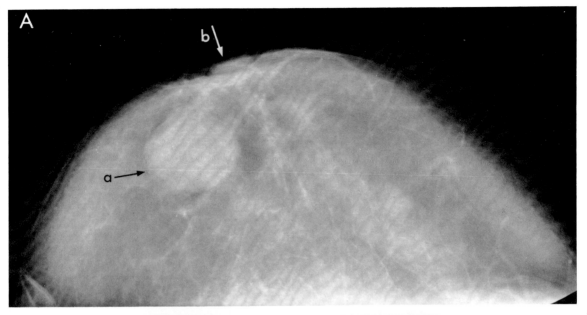

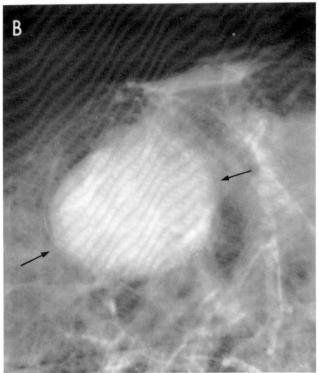

Figure 49 · Intraductal Papilloma / 111

Figure 50.—Gynecomastia.

Biopsy of a tender nodule beneath the right nipple of an 80-year-old man showed gynecomastia.

A, mediolateral view.

B, craniocaudal view.

The breast is enlarged and there is an irregular masslike density (**arrows**) beneath the nipple (**a**).

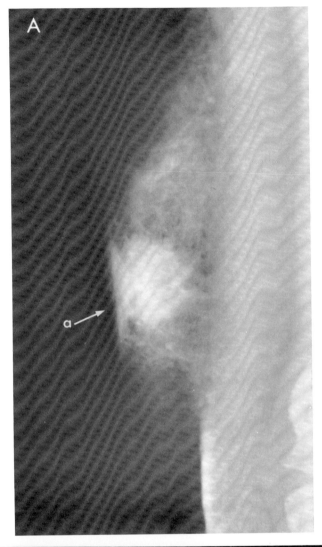

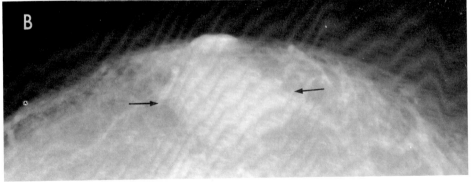

Figure 50 · Gynecomastia / 113

Figure 51.—Plasma cell mastitis.

Acute onset of pain and swelling of the breast of a 36-year-old multiparous woman occurred 4 weeks previously. The symptoms had subsided at the time of examination, but a firm subareolar mass attached to the skin persisted. Clinically, the lesion was thought to be carcinoma. Biopsy revealed plasma cell mastitis.

Craniocaudal view: The subareolar masslike lesion is opaque and, in this instance, fairly well circumscribed (**a**). Some thickening of the skin of the areola (**b**) is present, suggesting carcinoma.

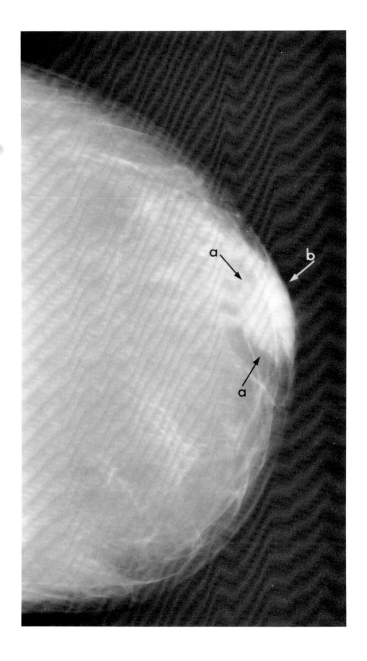

Figure 51 · Plasma Cell Mastitis / 115

Figure 52.—Mammary duct ectasia (comedomastitis).

A 59-year-old woman had a history of pain, tenderness and induration of the right breast. Palpable masses were present beneath both nipples, larger on the right. The nipples were retracted. Biopsy revealed mammary duct ectasia with subareolar fibrosis and calcification of the walls of the dilated ducts.

A, dense irregular fibrotic-appearing tissue (**a**) with nipple retraction (**b**) and coarse linear and ringlike calcifications (**c**) are seen.

A 72-year-old multiparous woman had a small palpable mass in the central portion of the right breast. There was no history of breast disease. The palpable nodule proved to be a small (1.5 cm) carcinoma, and the rest of the breast showed extensive mammary duct ectasia with calcifications in the walls of the ducts.

B, craniocaudal view: coarse linear and rounded calcifications are present throughout the breast. Little periductal and subareolar fibrosis is seen on the mammogram in this case. The small carcinoma (**a**) lies in the central portion of the breast and is partially obscured by a large collection of benign calcifications which overlie it.

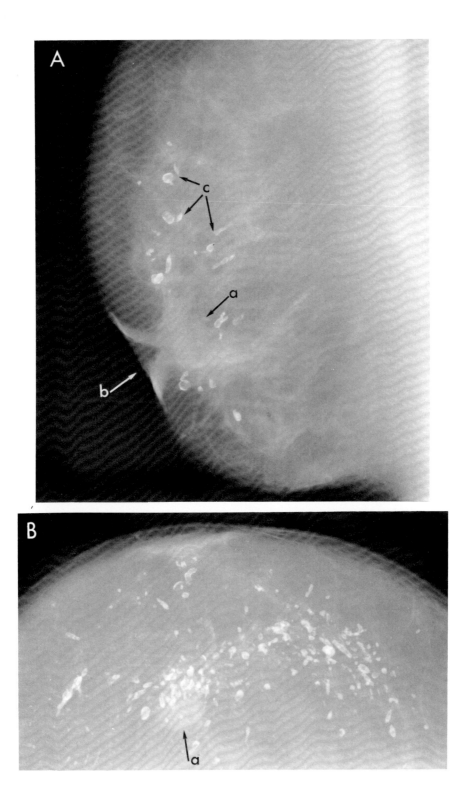

Figure 52 · Mammary Duct Ectasia / 117

Figure 53.—Galactocele.

A tender palpable mass in the right breast of a 34-year-old lactating woman developed during the fourth week after delivery. Biopsy revealed galactocele.

The radiolucent smooth-walled cystic-appearing mass (**arrows**), typical of galactocele, is seen in the central portion of the breast deep to the nipple. The radiopaque parenchyma of the lactating breast, surrounding the lesion, provides sharp contrast.

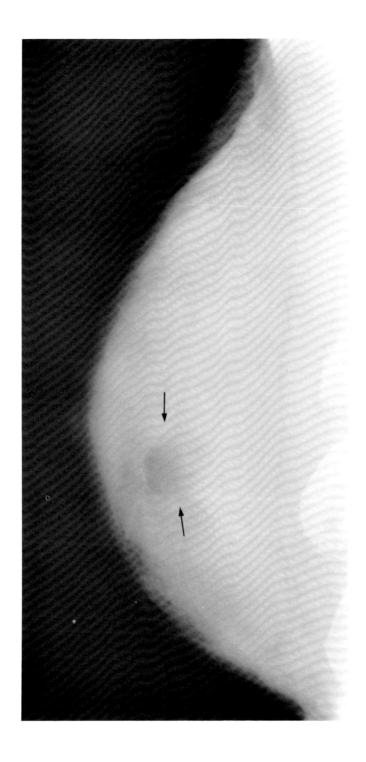

Figure 53 · Galactocele / 119

Figure 54.—Lipoma.

A prominent soft lobular mass was present in the right breast of a 60-year-old asymptomatic woman with large fatty breasts. Clinically and radiographically, the lesion was a lipoma, and biopsy was not done.

The fibrous wall of a large radiolucent lipoma is indicated by the **arrows.**

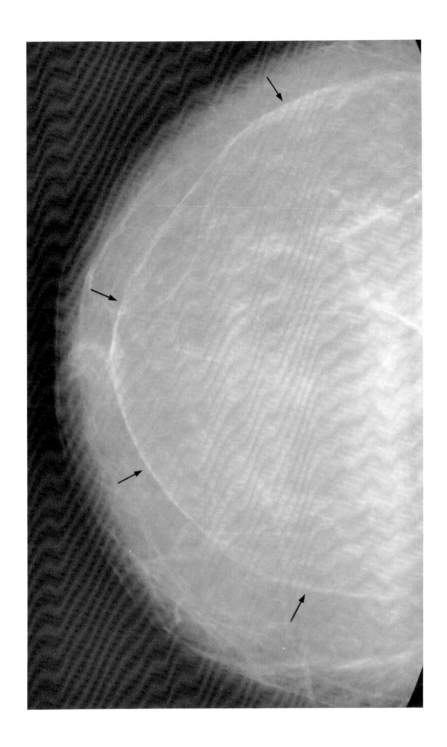

Figure 54 · Lipoma / 121

Figure 55.—Hematoma.

Examination of the breast of a 48-year-old woman, 2 weeks after excisional biopsy of a carcinoma by her home physician, showed that the skin incision was healed but that an irregular fluctuant mass was present at the operative site. A radical mastectomy was performed, and a 5 cm hematoma with a well-organized wall was found. There was no residual carcinoma.

The appearance of the large irregular mass (**arrows**) with prominent overlying veins suggests carcinoma. In most cases, a biopsy site, even when recent, is difficult to identify on the mammogram unless a hematoma develops, as in this case, or unless there is infection of the wound.

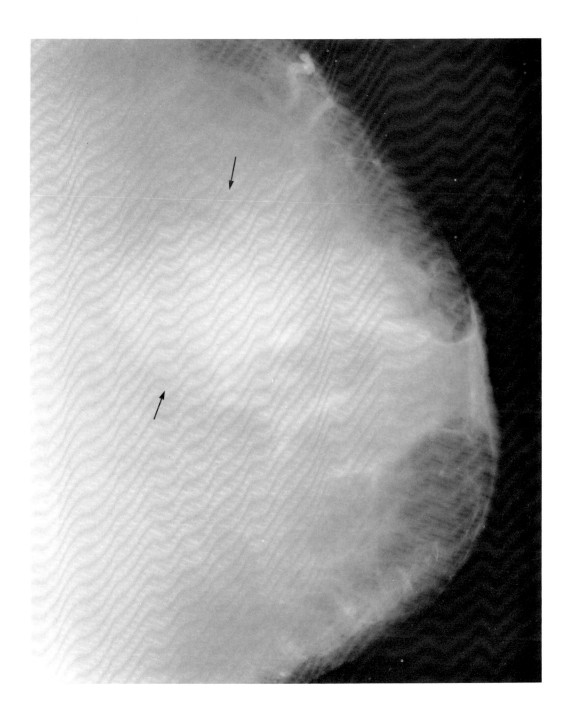

Figure 55 · Hematoma / 123

Figure 56.—Breast prosthesis; augmentation mammoplasty.

A 33-year-old woman had had an Ivalon-sponge prosthesis placed in the breast 2 years previously.

A, the prosthesis (**arrows**) presents as a sharply circumscribed radiopaque mass. No abnormality is seen in the adjacent breast tissue.

A hard palpable mass was present in the breast of a 30-year-old woman 3 years after augmentation mammoplasty involving the use of subcutaneous fat from the thigh.

B, a cystlike fatty structure (**arrows**) contains extensive calcification in its wall. The surrounding breast parenchyma appears normal.

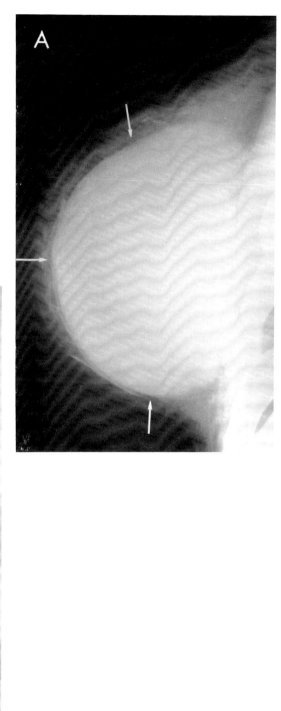

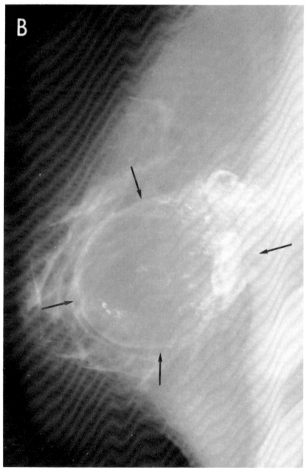

Figure 56 · Breast Prosthesis; Augmentation Mammoplasty / 125

Figure 57.—Benign tumors of the skin: nevus; keratosis; epidermoid cyst.

A, large, papillary nevus; craniocaudal view.

The lesion (**arrows**) is lobulated and its margins are sharply demarcated. If viewed at the proper angle, its attachment to the skin is seen. Nevi may be confused radiographically with benign intramammary tumors.

B, seborrheic keratosis; craniocaudal view.

The margins of this lesion (**arrow**) are irregular and it occasionally, as in this case, contains dense flecks suggesting calcification. It can at times be confused with a small carcinoma.

C, epidermoid cyst.

The lesion is sharply circumscribed, smooth walled and homogeneous. Its attachment to the skin can be seen (**a**). Unless infected, epidermoid cysts are easily distinguished from carcinoma.

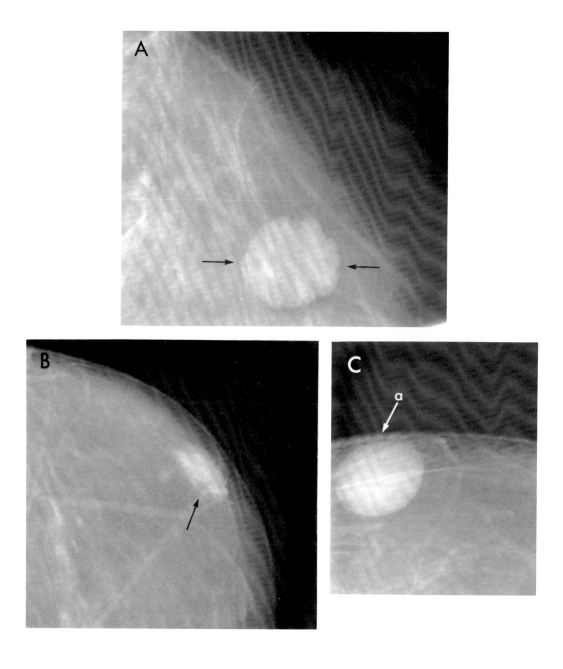

Figure 57 · Nevus; Keratosis; Epidermoid Cyst / 127

Figure 58.—Acute breast abscess.

A 36-year-old woman had a history of acute onset of pain, tenderness and swelling of the right breast. On examination, the central portion of the breast around the nipple was swollen, hot and tender. The process subsided under penicillin therapy, but a subareolar abscess developed and was drained. *Staphylococcus aureus* was cultured from the abscess.

A, right breast, craniocaudal view: Marked thickening of the skin of the nipple, areola and surrounding area (**a**) is present. The tissues deep to the nipple are opaque, and the architectural pattern of the subareolar portion of the breast is disrupted (**b**).

B, left breast, craniocaudal view: This view of the normal opposite breast is presented for comparison.

Case continued in Figure 59.

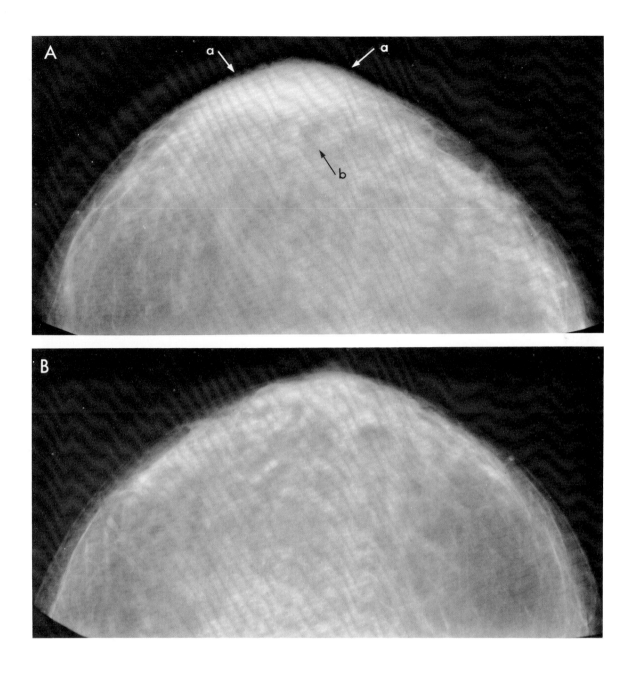

Figure 58 · Acute Breast Abscess / 129

Figure 59.—Acute breast abscess.

Mediolateral view: same case as Figure 58. The subareolar mass (**a**) accompanied by skin thickening (**b**) and increased vascularity (**c**) is well demonstrated.

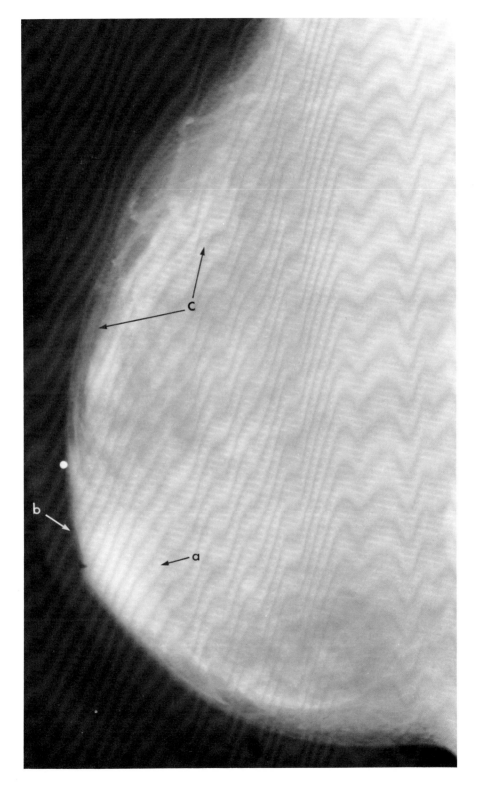

Figure 59 · Acute Breast Abscess / 131

Figure 60.—Acute inflammatory process of undetermined etiology.

A 78-year-old woman had a 2-week history of swelling, redness, tenderness and increased temperature of the right breast. Clinically, an acute inflammatory process could not be differentiated from diffuse inflammatory carcinoma. Biopsy demonstrated comedomastitis associated with an acute inflammatory process. No causative organism was cultured.

A, right breast, craniocaudal view.

B, left breast, craniocaudal view.

On the mamogram of the right breast (**A**) there are marked, diffuse thickening of the skin (**a**), increased vascularity (**b**), apparent nipple retraction (**c**) and what appears to be a large irregular mass filling most of the breast (**d**). No signs are present which differentiate inflammatory processes from diffuse inflammatory carcinoma in this case. Normal left breast (**B**) for comparison.

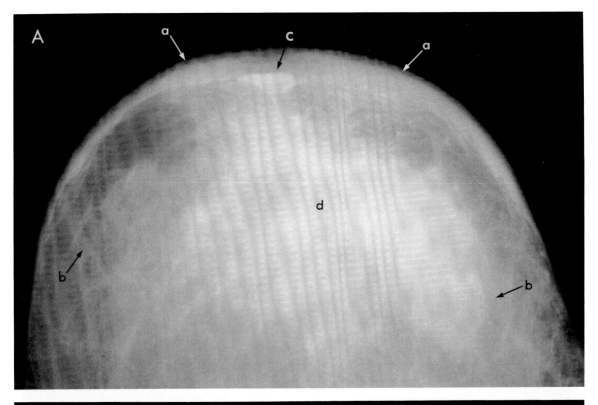

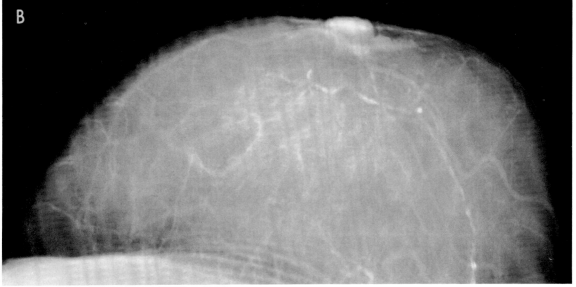

Figure 60 · Acute Inflammatory Process / 133

Figure 61.—Chronic inflammatory process with foreign body granuloma.

A 55-year-old woman had had six previous biopsies of the left breast because of fibrocystic disease. For 2 weeks she had had a mass, localized swelling and redness medial to the nipple. Clinically, the lesion appeared to be carcinoma. Excision of the region revealed chronic inflammatory changes with foci of foreign body, giant cell reaction and fibrosis associated with fragments of cotton fiber (old suture).

A, entire breast, craniocaudal view.

B, enlarged segment of the lesion, craniocaudal view: The mass is quite irregular and several rather coarse calcifications (**a**) are present within it. A localized area of thickened skin (**b**) overlies the lesion and extends to involve the areola. The appearance is entirely compatible with that of carcinoma.

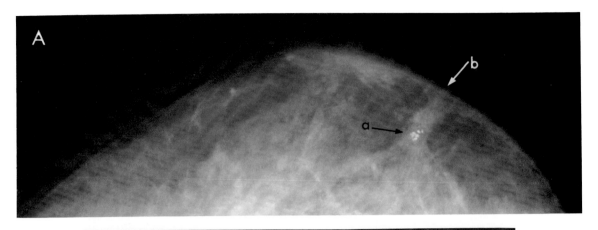

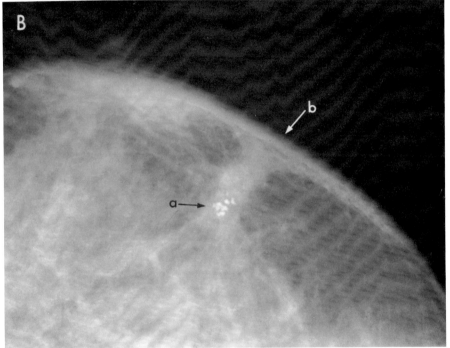

Figure 61 · Inflammation with Foreign Body Granuloma / 135

Figure 62.—Acute inflammatory disease—herpes zoster.

A 77-year-old woman gave a 5-day history of severe pain in the left lateral chest wall and left breast, associated with swelling, tenderness and cutaneous bleb formation. Clinically, the lesion was typical of acute herpes zoster. No biopsy was made.

On the mammogram, the diffuse thickening of the skin of the breast (**a**) mimics the appearance of diffuse carcinoma, and even though no mass is seen in the breast, malignant disease must be considered first on the basis of the mammographic appearance.

A wide variety of benign lesions will produce diffuse skin thickening in the breast which mimics that seen in diffuse or inflammatory carcinoma. Scleroderma, obstruction of the superior vena cava, pemphigus and lymphedema of unknown etiology are among the processes reported to cause this abnormality.

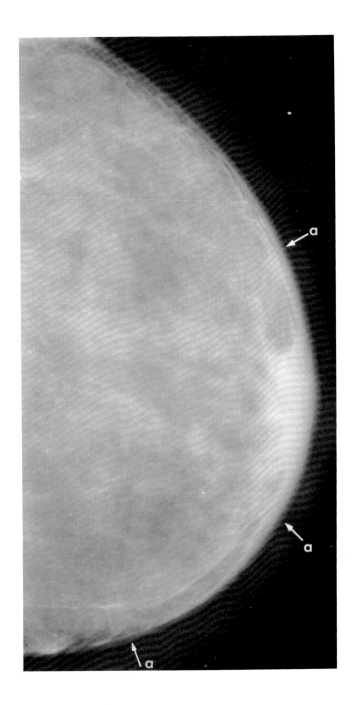

Figure 62 · Herpes Zoster / 137

CHAPTER 4

Malignant Tumors of the Breast

MALIGNANT TUMORS of the breast, like the benign tumors discussed in Chapter 3, present radiographic features which are, for the most part, characteristic and readily identified on the mammogram. These lesions in their classic forms are easily distinguished from benign disease by their irregular outline and by their tendencies to infiltrate surrounding structures, disrupt the normal architecture of the breast and destroy normal tissues. Others, however, are difficult to identify on the mammogram because they either are obscured by overlying radiopaque glandular tissues or are atypical in appearance. A few mimic benign disease. Many of these difficult or confusing cases are presented here alongside cases with characteristic radiographic findings of malignant disease, in order that the reader will be fully aware of the limitations of mammography as well as of its value in the detection and diagnosis of malignant tumors of the breast.

Roughly 98% of primary malignant tumors of the breast are adenocarcinomas. The various morphologic types of this disease as well as the rare primary sarcomas of the breast and metastases to the breast from primary tumors located elsewhere in the body present a broad spectrum of radiographic appearances that reflect the variations in pattern of growth seen among these tumors.

CARCINOMAS OF THE BREAST

INFILTRATING DUCTAL CARCINOMA WITH FIBROSIS

Infiltrating ductal carcinoma associated with greater or lesser amounts of fibrosis (synonyms and related terms: ordinary mammary scirrhous carcinoma, scirrhous carcinoma, carcinoma simplex, sclerosing carcinoma) is the common form of carcinoma found in the breast and from both a radiographic and pathologic standpoint is the type referred to in descriptions of the classic features of this disease.

Both direct (primary) and indirect (secondary) radiographic signs of malignant disease are seen on the mammogram. The *direct* signs are found in the appearance of the mass itself—its *shape, density,* the *character of its margins* and *its pattern of growth.* The *indirect* signs represent changes in the breast associated with or resulting from the presence of the tumor and include, among others, *calcification within the tumor, thickening of the skin, enlargement of veins* (increased vascularity), *retraction of the skin and nipple* and *abnormalities of the architectural pattern of the breast parenchyma.* None of the radiographic signs of malignant disease are pathognomonic, but many—including the calcifications found in the tumor and the irregular infiltrative appearance of some invasive carcinomas—are nearly so.

DIRECT (PRIMARY) SIGNS OF MALIGNANCY.—Variations in the pattern of growth of carcinoma and consequently the mammographic appearance of the carcinomatous mass are extreme. In its most common and characteristic forms (Figs. **63–68**), infiltrative ductal carcinoma of the scirrhous type presents the following classic radiographic characteristics:

1. Shape—irregularly rounded, discrete mass.
2. Density—variable, nonhomogeneous, more dense at the center than at the periphery.
3. Margins—irregular and indistinct, with spicules or tendrils of tumor radiating outward. This produces a "sunburst" appearance.
4. Pattern of growth—invasive and poorly circumscribed. This distorts and destroys the architectural pattern of normal surrounding tissues.

In other cases, the appearance ranges from a well-circumscribed nodular mass which may mimic benign disease such as cyst or fibroadenoma (Figs. **69–73**) through all types of irregular invasive patterns, with and without a well-formed tumor mass (Figs. **74–77**), to diffuse lesions with no definite mass and little or no radiographic abnormality to point to their presence (Figs. **78** and **79**).

Carcinoma arising in a subareolar location often presents special problems in diagnosis. As has been pointed out in Chapter 2, in the normal breast the subareolar region is usually occupied by radiopaque lactiferous ducts and periductal fibrous connective tissue. Subareolar fibrosis associated with mammary duct ectasia, plasma cell mastitis and other benign processes (Chap. 3) are also frequently seen. The opacity of the tissues in this region and the irregular fibrosis which is present in many cases tend to obliterate this radiographic evidence of carcinoma.

Typically, carcinoma in the subareolar area produces an irregular mass with stellate margins (Fig. **80**) like lesions located in deeper portions of the breast, but often (Figs. **81** and **82**) these signs are partially obscured and diagnosis is based on the presence of alterations in the architectural pattern, skin thickening, nipple retraction and tumor calcifications. All too frequently, carcinoma in this region is hidden by overlying benign disease (Fig. **83**).

INDIRECT (SECONDARY) SIGNS OF MALIGNANT DISEASE.—The indirect or secondary signs of malignant disease are abnormalities which represent changes in the breast associated with tumor, such as calcification, or abnormalities which result from the effects of tumor on the surrounding otherwise normal tissues, structures and landmarks. Among the latter group, thickening of the skin, distortion of the architectural pattern of the breast, enlargement of veins (increased vascularity) and retraction of the nipple and skin are the abnormalities most frequently seen. Direct invasion of the skin by tumor and obliteration of the retromammary space are occasionally observed.

The wide variation in appearance of carcinoma and the frequent occurrence of carcinoma in radiopaque glandular breasts often make it difficult to recognize the disease from the appearance of the mass alone. In these cases, the indirect signs of malignant tumor are as important to diagnosis as is the appearance of the tumor itself. In fact, one finds in practice that there are many instances in which the secondary signs produce the only radiographic evidence of malignant tumor.

Calcification in carcinoma.—Deposits of calcium are demonstrated on the mammogram in roughly one third of the cases of carcinoma of the breast and can be detected on histologic study of specimens in 60–75% of the cases. These are most often formed within necrotic regions in intraductal carcinoma. This holds even in those cases which are predominantly of the scirrhous type.[1]

In contrast to the calcifications found in benign disease (see Chap. 3, Figs. 27, 42 and 52), which tend to be rounded, few in number, coarse, relatively uniform in size and widely scattered, the calcifications in carcinoma are typically irregular in outline, variable in size and numerous (Fig. **84**). They are localized to the region of the tumor, but some appear outside the primary mass itself and on microscopic examination are found in tumor-filled ducts extending away from the main body of the lesion (Figs. **85** and **86**). Occasionally, they are arranged in a linear fashion along a single duct or duct system (Fig. **87**). It is a characteristic of malignant calcifications that the more carefully one looks at the mammogram the more calcification

[1] Levitan, L. H.; Witten, D. M., and Harrison, E. G., Jr.: Am. J. Roentgenol. 92:29, 1964.

one sees, but in some instances only a few rather coarse calcifications are present (Fig. **88**). These are difficult to distinguish from calcifications of benign disease.

The calcifications of the malignant type illustrated here are of great importance to diagnosis, especially when opaque overlying tissues obscure the mass or when the tumor does not produce an identifiable mass on the mammogram (Figs. **89** and **90**). It is of equal importance to recognize that these calcifications, while characteristic of carcinoma, are not pathognomonic and that in a number of benign diseases, for example, sclerosing adenosis, ductal papillomatosis and fibrocystic disease, calcifications are occasionally found which are indistinguishable on the mammogram from those of carcinoma (Fig. **91**).

Thickening of the skin.—Thickening of the skin is a frequent and characteristic secondary sign of carcinoma. The process may be localized or diffuse. It is recognized clinically as localized deformity and thickening of the skin over the tumor in its early or localized stage (Fig. **92**), as thickening and induration of the skin of all or a large part of the breast in diffuse carcinoma (Figs. **93** and **94**) or as the classic "peau d'orange" of inflammatory carcinoma (Fig. **95**). This abnormality is ordinarily associated with lymphatic obstruction, but direct invasion by tumor is sometimes seen.

Disruption and distortion of the architectural pattern of the parenchyma of the breast ordinarily accompanies diffuse and inflammatory carcinoma. This takes the form of an increased opacity of the breast, loss of the normal orientation of ductal markings toward the nipple and obliteration of the subcutaneous fat line with dilatation of the subdermal lymphatics.

Enlargement of mammary veins (increased vascularity).—Unilateral enlargement of the mammary veins is found in rare instances in normal women and frequently with benign inflammatory disease and with carcinoma. In the presence of carcinoma it is thought to result from a localized increase in cellular metabolism in the growing tumor. Careful inspection of the mammogram and comparison of the size of comparable veins on the two sides is necessary to detect its presence.[2]

Since enlargement of veins is frequently found with benign lesions, it is not as reliable an indicator of the presence of carcinoma as is calcification, for example, but in some instances it is helpful in diagnosis and may lead the examiner to find a carcinoma which would otherwise be overlooked (Figs. **96–98**).

Retraction of skin and nipple; ulceration of skin.—Retraction of the skin and nipple results from shortening and thickening of the suspensory

[2] Dodd, G. D., and Wallace, J. D.: Radiology 90:900, 1968.

ligaments of the breast due to invasion by tumor and associated fibrosis. Retraction of the nipple is commonly seen when the tumor arises in the subareolar location (Fig. **99**) or when it is large and extends into the tissues beneath the nipple.

Retraction of the nipple may occur as a congenital abnormality (Fig. **100**), and it may be associated with benign diseases, such as mammary duct ectasia, when extensive subareolar fibrosis is present.

Retraction of the skin is seen clinically as "flattening" or "dimpling" of the skin over a tumor and is one of the characteristic clinical and radiographic signs of carcinoma (Fig. **101**).

Extension of tumor through the skin to form an ulcerated mass represents a far-advanced stage of disease. Lesions which have reached this advanced stage of growth are rare in most practices today (Fig. **102**).

Obliteration of the retromammary space.—Obliteration of the retromammary space as the result of extension of tumor into the pectoral muscles and anterior chest wall (Fig. **103**) is uncommon, but when it is seen, it may be of some assistance to the surgeon in planning his operation. Demonstration of this process requires careful positioning of the patient for the mediolateral projection to show the retromammary space to best advantage (see Chap. 2, Fig. 10).

Axillary lymphadenopathy.—Demonstration of axillary lymph nodes by means of conventional mammographic technique is difficult and seldom contributes to the care of the patient. Examination of the axilla, with its thick radiopaque tissues, requires the use of higher energy x-rays than are used for examination of the breast itself, and as a consequence the radiographic contrast of the axillary tissues is greatly reduced. Because of this reduction in contrast, small lymph nodes are not visible, and in ordinary circumstances, only grossly enlarged nodes can be identified (Figs. **104** and **105**). These are seen as well-circumscribed densities which appear the same whether enlarged by metastatic tumor, lymphoma or inflammation. In very rare cases, calcifications in metastases from carcinoma of the breast can be identified (Fig. **106**).

COMEDOCARCINOMA

The term comedocarcinoma is used to describe carcinoma that arises in the mammary ducts and forms solid plugs of tumor in the ducts. This lesion is found in both noninfiltrating (Figs. **107** and **108**) and infiltrating (Figs. **109–112**) stages of growth. It occurs in a mixed form with other types of infiltrative duct carcinoma in most instances, but it is the predominate morphologic type in 5–10% of the cases.

Radiographically, the most important feature of this type of tumor is calcification. In my experience, this lesion has contained mammographically identifiable calcifications in approximately three fourths of the cases, and typical punctate tumor calcifications, such as those seen in scirrhous-type carcinoma, are almost invariably located in areas of comedocarcinoma mixed in the predominantly scirrhous lesion. Aside from the tendency to form calcifications and a tendency to produce a diffuse, poorly circumscribed tumor, comedocarcinoma has no features which distinguish it from other types of carcinoma.

PAPILLARY CARCINOMA

Papillary carcinoma in a relatively pure form is a rare histologic type of ductal carcinoma. It is characterized by malignant papillary ingrowths into the mammary ducts and, in the invasive form, by infiltration by tumor with maintenance of the basic papillary structure. More frequently, it is seen in mixed lesions, with comedo, fibrotic or lobular histologic patterns predominating. Bloody nipple discharge is a frequent complaint. Both noninfiltrating (Fig. 113) and infiltrating (Figs. 114 and 115) forms are seen.

Radiographically, calcification is usually not a prominent feature, although it can occur. The tumor may form a discrete well-circumscribed mass, but in many instances it produces a multinodular appearance which suggests comedomastitis or fibrocystic disease. In most instances, the radiographic diagnosis of malignant tumor is difficult.

MEDULLARY CARCINOMA

Medullary carcinoma with lymphoid stroma produces a large bulky tumor which in most cases is well circumscribed and even when quite large does not have clinical signs such as fixation and skin dimpling which are commonly associated with carcinoma. Many of these lesions are partially cystic, and hemorrhage and necrosis are common.

On the mammogram, medullary carcinoma usually appears as a well-circumscribed mass (Fig. 116). Calcification within the tumor is uncommon, and in most cases, evidence of invasion of surrounding tissues is difficult to detect. In rare instances, medullary carcinoma does not form a bulky well-circumscribed mass but instead assumes a more diffuse pattern of growth (Fig. 117).

COLLOID (MUCINOUS) CARCINOMA

Mucin production is frequently observed in infiltrative ductal carcinomas of all types, and the usage of the terms "colloid carcinoma" and "mucinous carcinoma" varies widely. As a rule, however, these terms are used to describe tumors in which the production of mucinous material is highly developed and a dominant characteristic of the lesion.

In most instances, when mucin is present in large quantity, the tumor assumes a circumscribed appearance with sharply demarcated margins and a homogeneous density. However, close scrutiny of the margins of the tumor reveals evidence of the infiltrative nature of the lesion (Figs. **118** and **119**). In some cases, the tumor is poorly circumscribed and has irregular invasive margins (Fig. **120**). Calcification is rare in this disease, but when seen, the calcifications are large, irregular and dense and do not have the extreme variation in size seen in the more common types of tumor calcification (Fig. **121**).

LOBULAR CARCINOMA

Lobular carcinoma is an uncommon morphologic type of breast cancer which makes up less than 5% of cases in most series. Both noninfiltrating and infiltrating forms are recognized. The noninfiltrating or in situ form involves the lobular ducts and acini. It is often bilateral and is difficult to detect clinically. Since the advent of mammography, however, it is detected with increasing frequency.[3] Minute calcifications in the form of localized areas of punctate or linear flecks are the most characteristic mammographic findings (Fig. **122**), but in some instances, a poorly marginated area of localized density is seen. In others, no radiographic abnormality is present.

Infiltrating lobular carcinoma is rarely seen in a pure state, but it is seen often in mixed lesions, in association with lobular, comedo, papillary and scirrhous elements. Both clinically and radiographically this lesion resembles the ordinary forms of carcinoma (Figs. **123** and **124**).

PAGET'S DISEASE

Paget's disease is an eczematoid change in the nipple and areola of the breast resulting from invasion of the skin by carcinoma arising in the main excretory ducts of the breast. The lesion is characterized histologically by invasion of the epidermis by large anaplastic cells known as Paget cells. The underlying carcinoma may be small and difficult to demonstrate.

---

[3] Snyder, R. E.: Surg., Gynec. & Obst. 122:255, 1966.

On the mammogram, the most frequent finding is a slight thickening of the skin of the nipple and areola (Fig. **125**). This change is often so subtle that it is overlooked unless the examiner is aware that clinical signs suggesting Paget's disease are present. In other cases, the underlying carcinoma can be identified, and when seen, it may contain flecks of calcium (Fig. **126**).

INTRACYSTIC CARCINOMA

Intracystic carcinoma is a rare form of mammary tumor in which an infiltrating, usually papillary, tumor is present in the wall of a cyst. Even when the tumor is large, a portion of the cyst wall is not involved in the malignant process. On the mammogram, these tumors appear well circumscribed and often mimic benign lesions. Usually, however, evidence of tumor infiltration is seen on the side of the cyst occupied by the tumor. Fine calcifications are occasionally present (Figs. **127** and **128**).

APOCRINE "SWEAT GLAND" CARCINOMA

Apocrine sweat gland carcinomas are rare lesions which comprise 1% or less of carcinomas of the breast. Histologically, the predominant cells resemble those of the cutaneous apocrine sweat glands. These give the lesion its name. There are no gross morphologic or radiographic features which distinguish this lesion from other types of adenocarcinoma of the breast. The few examples of this disease that I have studied have been diffusely infiltrative lesions (Fig. **129**).

ADENOID CYSTIC CARCINOMA

Adenoid cystic carcinoma (cylindroma) of the breast is histologically indistinguishable from similar lesions of the salivary glands, trachea and bronchi. Only two examples of this lesion were encountered among 1,100 carcinomas studied with mammography by the author. The lesion is so rare that no generalizations can be made concerning its radiographic appearance, but both of our tumors were in breasts of elderly patients and produced an irregular lesion with an indistinct, poorly marginated outline. The appearance of both tumors suggested thickening of ductal structures (Fig. **130**).

UNCOMMON MANIFESTATIONS

MULTICENTRIC CARCINOMA.—There is a strong tendency toward multicentric origin of carcinomas of the breast. This is seen with greatest frequency in comedo, papillary and lobular forms where multicentric origin is often observed along a single duct or in many ducts throughout the breast (see Figs. 84, 110, 115, and 124). Occasionally, multiple carcinomas of the same histologic pattern (Fig. **131**) and even two or more carcinomas of different histologic patterns (Fig. **132**) develop simultaneously in different parts of the breast. Aside from the presence of two or more tumors in the breast, these lesions have no clinical or radiologic characteristics which distinguish them from the ordinary solitary carcinoma.

SIMULTANEOUS BILATERAL CARCINOMA.—Simultaneous bilateral carcinoma is uncommon. In most series in which mammography has not been part of the preoperative examination, it is found in less than 1% of the cases. With preoperative mammography, however, there appears to be a substantial increase in the number of such lesions detected. Most appear to be separate primary tumors which are often of different cell types (Figs. **133** and **134**). The importance of removal of both lesions is obvious since either may metastasize and cause the death of the patient.

CARCINOMA OF THE REMAINING BREAST FOLLOWING MASTECTOMY.— A second carcinoma develops in the remaining breast at some time after unilateral mastectomy in from 7 to 9% or more of the cases. Some are metastases which may be either diffuse or localized (Figs. **135** and **136**). New primary tumors are common, however, and may in fact be more prevalent than metastases (Figs. **137** and **138**). Mammography is of considerable assistance in detection of these tumors while they are still at an early stage of growth.

CARCINOMA OF BREAST DURING PREGNANCY.—Carcinoma of the breast which arises during pregnancy presents a difficult diagnostic problem to both the clinician and the mammographer. In an occasional case, a typical infiltrating carcinoma is seen (Fig. **139**). In other cases, a lesion can be identified but because of the density of the overlying glandular tissues, its margins cannot be seen with enough clarity for diagnosis (Fig. **140**). In the large majority of cases, the glandular tissues are dense, totally obscuring the carcinoma, and the presence of a lesion can only be suspected when secondary signs such as skin thickening (Fig. **141**) develop.

CARCINOMA OF THE MALE BREAST.—Carcinoma of the male breast is infrequent, occurring in a proportion of about 1:100, as compared to carcinoma of the female breast. On the mammogram, these lesions ordinarily present the same radiographic characteristics as carcinoma of the female breast (Figs. **142** and **143**), but occasionally they are difficult to distinguish from gynecomastia (Fig. **144**).

LYMPHOMA OF THE BREAST

Lymphoma of the breast is rarely seen as a primary lesion but rather is usually a manifestation of generalized disease. On the mammogram, these tumors have no features that distinguish them from the more circumscribed or diffuse carcinomas. These lesions may occur as discrete circumscribed masses in the breast (Fig. **145**), as diffusely infiltrating tumors involving the entire breast (Fig. **146**) or as masses of enlarged axillary lymph nodes (Fig. **147**). Thickening of the skin of the breast due to lymphatic obstruction by lymphoma in the axillary and cervical lymph nodes is occasionally observed (Fig. **148**).

MISCELLANEOUS SARCOMAS OF THE BREAST

The various sarcomas are for the most part pathologic and radiographic curiosities which comprise an almost vanishingly small proportion of the malignant tumors affecting the breast. Because of their rarity, no generalizations as to their radiographic characteristics are possible. Primary and metastatic melanoma are illustrated by Figures **149** and **150,** respectively; angiosarcoma by Figure **151,** and rhabdomyosarcoma by Figure **152.** All present as well-circumscribed lesions which are difficult to distinguish from benign tumors. In addition to these types, I have observed two cases of liposarcoma, both of which were radiolucent fatty masses which were not radiographically different from benign lipoma.

Figure 63.—Scirrhous carcinoma: typical radiographic features.

A 66-year-old woman had a hard, palpable mass in the midportion of the right breast. The clinical diagnosis was carcinoma, and a radical mastectomy was performed. Pathologically, the lesion was a grade 3 adenocarcinoma of the scirrhous type, 4 cm in diameter. Three lymph nodes low in the right axilla contained metastatic carcinoma.

Mammogram, craniocaudal view: The tumor (**arrow**) is irregularly rounded and very opaque as contrasted with the surrounding fatty-type breast tissue. The density is not uniform throughout the mass but is greater in the center than at the periphery. The margins are irregular and poorly circumscribed. Fine spicules of tumor invade the surrounding normal breast tissue, giving a typical sunburst appearance.

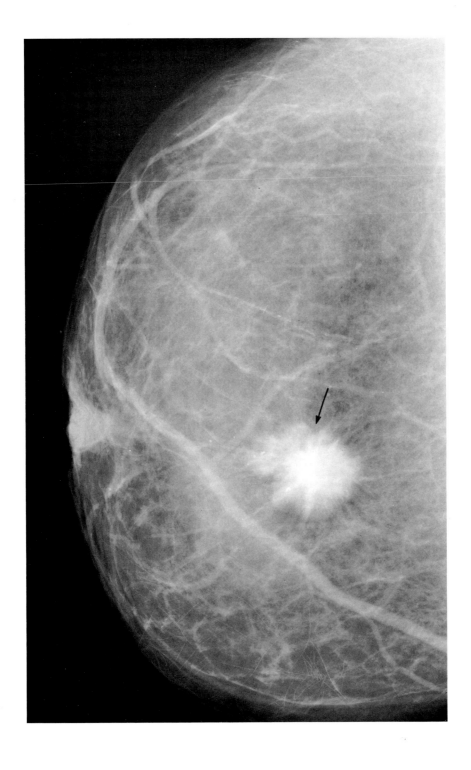

Figure 63 · Scirrhous Carcinoma—Radiographic Features / 149

Figure 64.—Typical scirrhous carcinoma: variations in appearance of margin.

A, circumscribed form—fine spiculation.

B, circumscribed form—moderate spiculation.

C, noncircumscribed form—coarse, irregular spiculation. This is a radiograph of a section (1 cm thick) of a gross specimen.

Comment: The spicules or tendrils of tumor (**arrows**) invading surrounding normal breast tissue are the most characteristic features of carcinoma that are seen on the mammogram. The invading strands of tumor radiate at all angles from the mass and, in most instances, do not follow the normal architectural pattern of the ductal system toward the nipple.

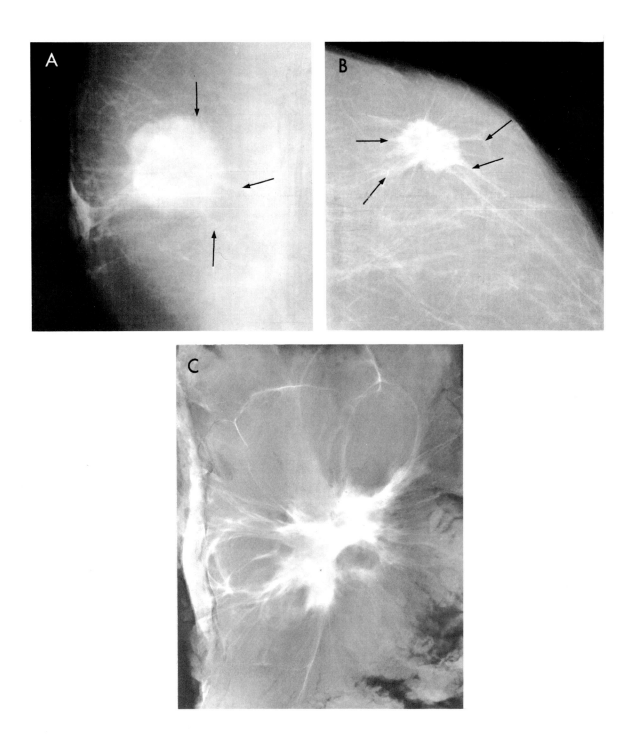

Figure 64 · Scirrhous Carcinoma—Variations of Margin / 151

Figure 65.—Typical scirrhous carcinoma with extension toward nipple.

A, carcinoma high in the upper outer quadrant of the right breast with a long thin spicule of tumor extending along the ductal system toward the nipple (**arrows**).

B, carcinoma in the central portion of the breast with extension to the nipple and thickening of the subareolar ducts (**arrows**).

Comment: In most instances, the invading strands of tumor radiate at all angles from the mass, disrupting the architectural pattern. In instances such as these, however, extensions of tumor along the ductal system toward the nipple distort and straighten the pattern of the normal mammary ducts.

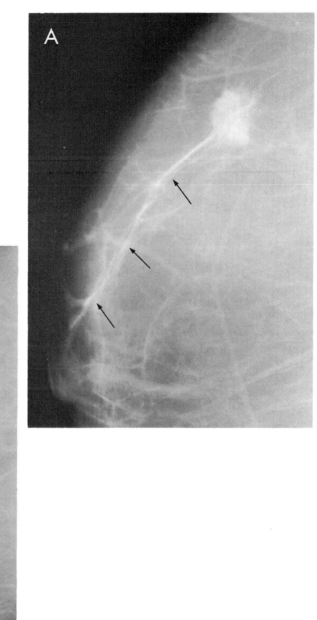

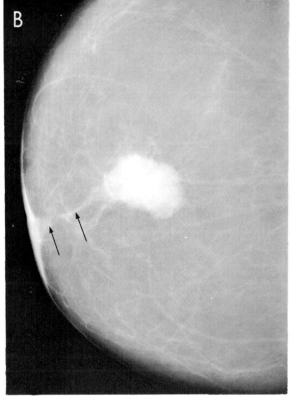

Figure 65 · Scirrhous Carcinoma: Extension toward Nipple / 153

Figure 66.—Carcinoma with extension toward axilla and base of breast—"comet" sign.

Craniocaudal view made with film holder shaped to conform to the contour of the chest wall: There is a poorly circumscribed scirrhous carcinoma (**a**) with a tail of tumor (**b**) growing posteriorly toward the chest wall, forming the so-called comet sign.

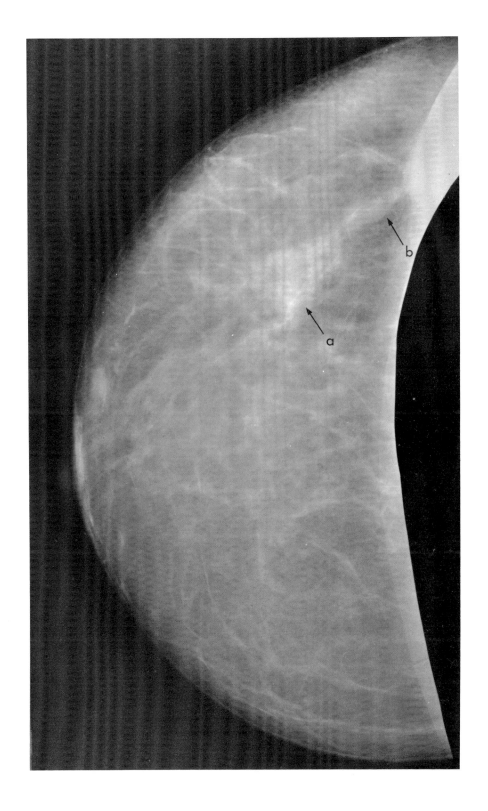

Figure 66 · Scirrhous Carcinoma: Comet Sign / 155

Figure 67.—Scirrhous carcinoma: disruption of architectural pattern of breast.

A 48-year-old woman who was menstruating regularly had no history of prior breast disease. A firm mass was palpable in the right breast, with diffuse nodularity throughout the remainder of the breast. A radical mastectomy was performed. Pathologically, the lesion was a scirrhous adenocarcinoma, 5 cm in diameter, in the central portion of the breast. Multiple axillary lymph nodes were involved by metastatic tumor.

A, right breast, mediolateral view: The carcinoma in the central portion of the breast is largely obscured by dense overlying glandular tissue. The normal architectural pattern of the breast is disrupted by the spiculated tumor (**arrows**), however, so that the lesion is easily recognized.

B, left breast, mediolateral view: Normal breast shown for comparison.

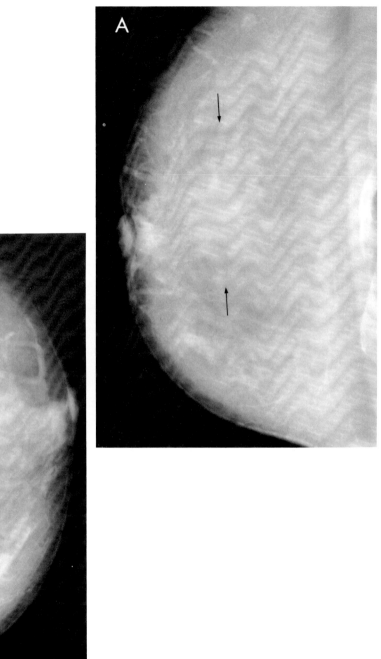

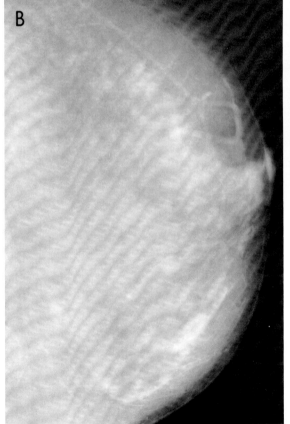

Figure 67 · Scirrhous Carcinoma: Disruption of Architecture / 157

Figure 68.—Scirrhous carcinoma: variations in appearance with size.

A, mammogram, craniocaudal view: Large (7 cm) scirrhous adenocarcinoma in the central portion of the breast is irregular and nonhomogeneous, though very dense. It has a spiculated margin typical of carcinoma.

B, mammogram, localized view: Tiny (0.8 mm) scirrhous adenocarcinoma (**arrow**) in the upper outer quadrant of the breast exhibits the same radiographic characteristics as does the large lesion. It is dense and stands out clearly in the fatty breast. The margins are irregular and spiculated and even at this small size produce a sunburst effect.

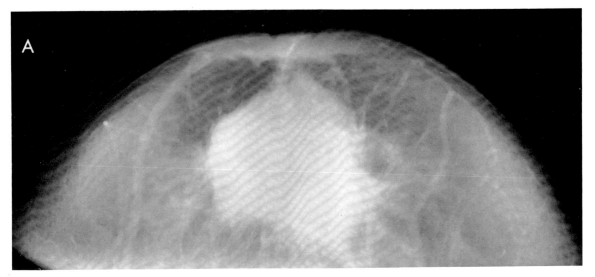

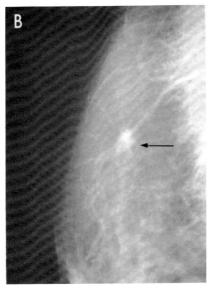

Figure 68 · Scirrhous Carcinoma: Variable Appearance with Size / 159

Figure 69.—Circumscribed carcinoma.

A 58-year-old woman had a mass in the medial aspect of the right breast. A radical mastectomy was performed. Pathologically, the lesion was a grade 4 adenocarcinoma, 2 cm in diameter. The axillary lymph nodes were free from metastatic tumor.

Mammogram, craniocaudal view: The well-circumscribed mass is lobular, is nonhomogeneous and has indistinct margins, especially on the posterior aspect (**a**), suggesting malignant disease. A tiny benign nodule (**b**) is present in the medial aspect of the breast. In many instances such as this, close scrutiny of the margins of the mass is required to detect evidence of invasive tumor.

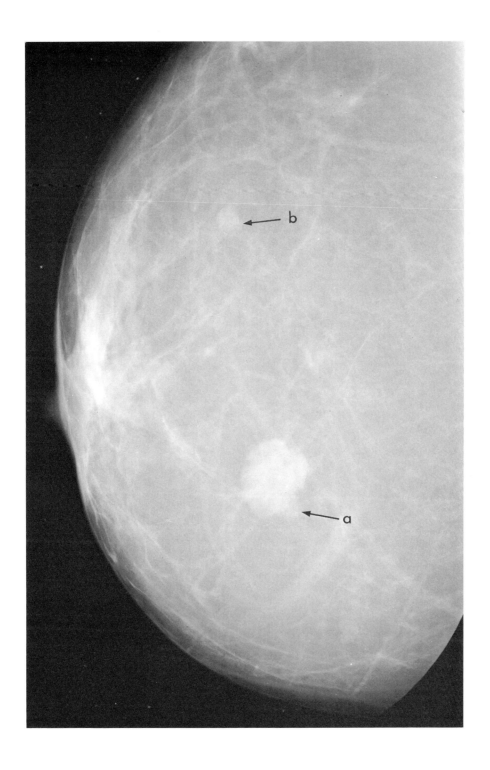

Figure 69 · Circumscribed Carcinoma / 161

Figure 70.—Circumscribed carcinoma.

A, mammogram, localized view: Most of the margin of this circumscribed grade 4 scirrhous carcinoma is well defined and smooth, but superiorly the margin is irregular and spiculated (**arrows**).

B, mammogram, mediolateral view: A circumscribed grade 3 scirrhous carcinoma in the upper portion of the right breast (**a**). The breast is moderately nodular and opaque due to the presence of fibrocystic changes. The larger portion of the tumor is very well circumscribed. It contains coarse rounded calcifications and is homogeneous in density, suggesting a benign cyst. On the posterior wall (**arrow**), however, invasive tumor is seen, which identifies the lesion as malignant.

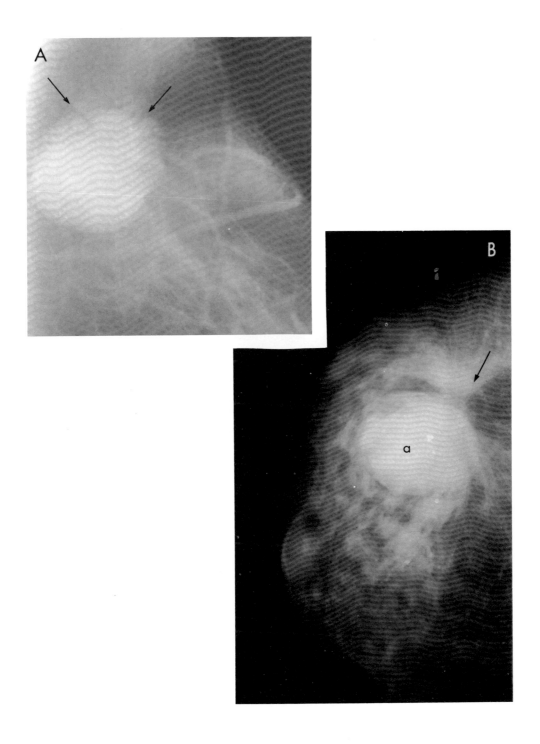

Figure 70 · Circumscribed Carcinoma / 163

Figure 71.—Circumscribed carcinoma: value of multiple views.

A 63-year-old woman had "thickening" and a possible mass in the axillary tail of the right breast on palpation. A radical mastectomy was performed. Pathologically, the lesion was a grade 4 scirrhous adenocarcinoma, 1 cm in diameter. One axillary node was involved by metastatic tumor.

A, mammogram, craniocaudal view: The tumor is not seen in the film because of its location high in the tail of the breast. The normal nipple (**arrow**) is not projected in profile.

B, upper part of mediolateral view: A well-circumscribed nodule is seen in the tail of the breast (**arrow**), but it is partially obscured by overlying fibrotic breast tissue (**a**) and its nature is not clearly evident.

C, compression spot view: The lesion is now clearly demonstrated. Although it is a circumscribed lesion, the margins are finely spiculated, indicating its malignant nature.

Comment: This case illustrates the value of multiple views of the breast for localization of a lesion and demonstration of its radiographic characteristics to best advantage.

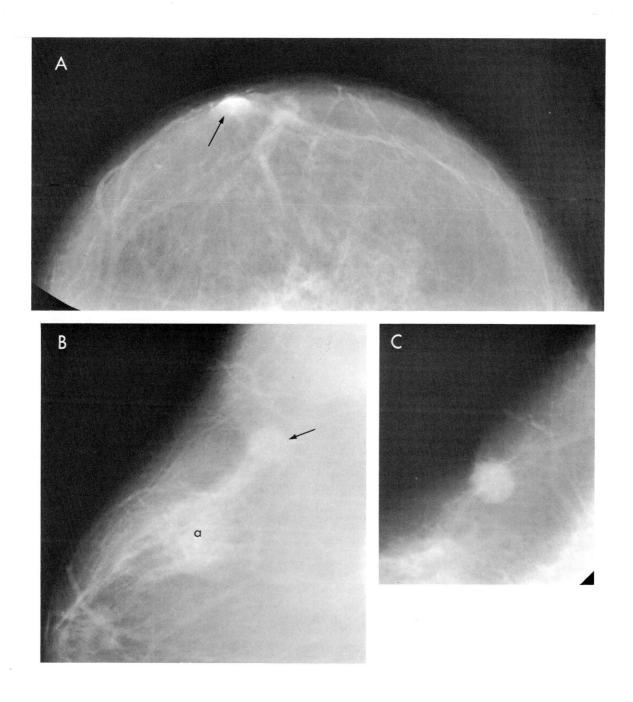

Figure 71 · Circumscribed Carcinoma: Multiple Views / 165

Figure 72.—Circumscribed carcinoma with cystic degeneration.

A 52-year-old multiparous woman had a large mass in the lateral aspect of the right breast. A radical mastectomy was performed. Pathologically, the lesion was a carcinoma, 5 × 5 × 3 cm. Within the tumor were three degenerative cysts containing necrotic material. Multiple small invasive nodules as well as several ducts filled with noninvasive carcinoma were present. The invasive nodules were of the "knobby" type.*

Mammogram, mediolateral view: There is a multinodular lesion with the margins of several of the nodules so sharply defined that they appear to be cysts (**a**). They are in direct continuity with ill-defined masses whose borders fade into the surrounding tissues (**b**). This appearance suggests the malignant nature of the lesion.

Figure 72, courtesy of Dr. J. E. Martin and Dr. H. S. Gallager, The University of Texas, M. D. Anderson Hospital and Tumor Institute, Houston.

* Gallagher, H. S., and Martin, J. E.: Cancer 23:855, 1969.

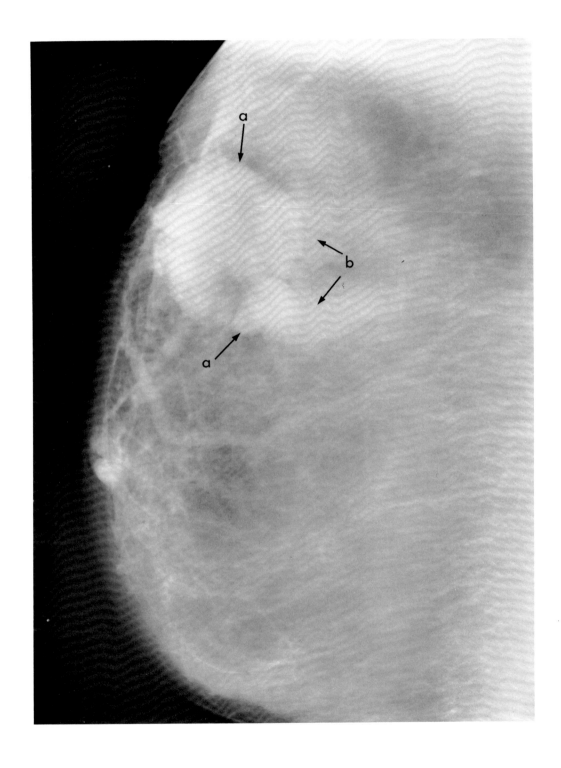

Figure 72 · Circumscribed Carcinoma: Cystic Degeneration / 167

Figure 73.—Circumscribed carcinoma mimicking benign tumor.

A 70-year-old woman had a firm, movable mass in the medial aspect of the left breast. A radical mastectomy was performed. Pathologically, the lesion was an encapsulated grade 4 adenocarcinoma, 3 cm in diameter. Axillary lymph nodes were free from tumor.

Mammogram, craniocaudal view: The sharply circumscribed lobular mass (**arrow**) has a homogeneous density, and there is no radiographic evidence of invasion of surrounding tissues. The lesion mimics a benign tumor such as fibroadenoma.

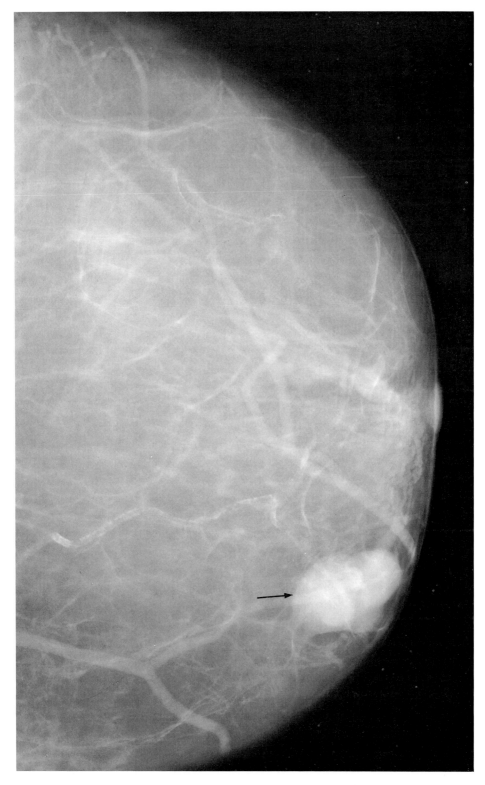

Figure 73 · Circumscribed Carcinoma: Mimicking Benign Tumor / 169

Figure 74.—Carcinoma with invasive pattern involving central portion of the breast.

A 67-year-old woman had had a mass palpable in the left breast for 5 months. Radical mastectomy was performed. Pathologically, the lesion comprised mixed scirrhous and mucus-producing adenocarcinoma involving the central portion of the breast and extending to involve the nipple. There were metastases to multiple axillary lymph nodes.

Mammogram, craniocaudal view: A large invasive carcinoma in the central portion of the breast (**a**) is associated with nipple retraction (**b**) and enlargement of the veins (**c**) due to increased blood flow in the breast.

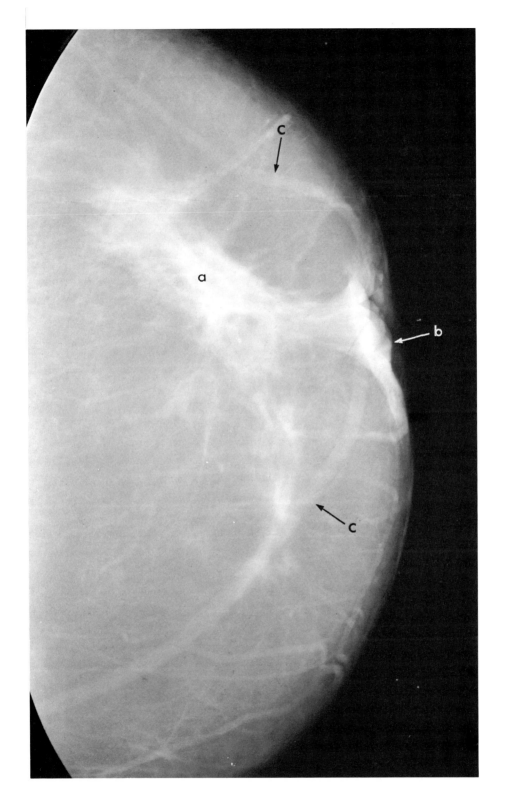

Figure 74 · Carcinoma: Invasive Pattern / 171

Figure 75.—Carcinoma with invasive pattern and a well-defined mass.

A 71-year-old woman had mammography for evaluation of nodularity in the right breast thought clinically to be benign. No mass was palpated in the left breast at physical examination. Carcinoma of the left breast was diagnosed by mammography. Left radical mastectomy was performed. Pathologically, the lesion was a grade 3 scirrhous adenocarcinoma, $4 \times 3 \times 2$ cm. Axillary lymph nodes were free from tumor.

Mammogram, craniocaudal view: The typical irregular carcinoma (**x**) has an invasive pattern of growth. Some flattening and thickening of the skin around the nipple is present (**arrow**).

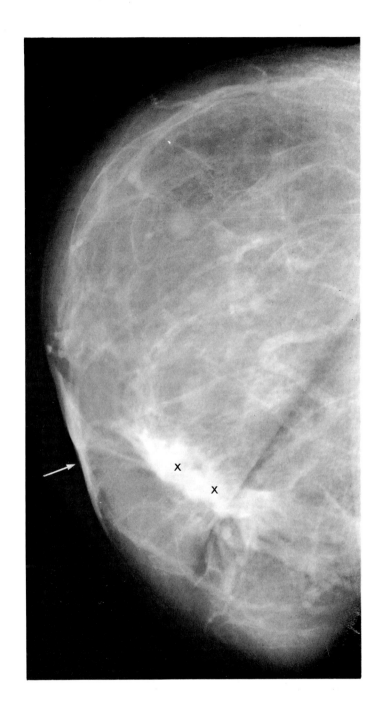

Figure 75 · Carcinoma: Invasive Pattern / 173

Figure 76.—Carcinoma with invasive pattern associated with diffuse fibrocystic disease.

A 64-year-old woman had a long history of fibrocystic disease. She had first noticed a palpable mass in the upper outer quadrant of the right breast 4 months previously. Clinically, this was carcinoma. Right radical mastectomy was performed. Pathologically, the irregular lesion was invasive grade 4 adenocarcinoma, 3.5 cm in greatest diameter, associated with diffuse fibrocystic disease. Multiple axillary lymph nodes were metastatically involved.

Mammogram, mediolateral view: The irregular tumor mass (**a**) blends into and is partially obscured by dense fibrotic breast tissue. Prominent irregular veins are seen in the region of the tumor. Note that the lesion does not extend through the retromammary space.

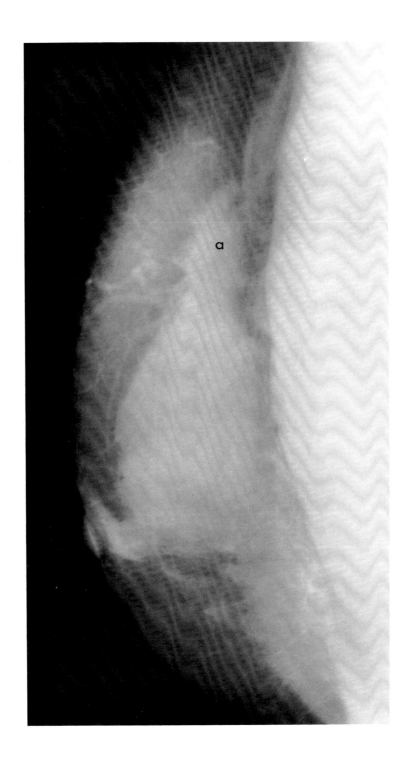

Figure 76 · Carcinoma: With Fibrocystic Disease / 175

Figure 77.—Carcinoma with invasive pattern and poorly defined mass.

A 59-year-old woman had a palpable mass in the left breast, first noticed 3 weeks previously. Radical mastectomy was performed. Pathologically, the lesion was a grade 3 scirrhous adenocarcinoma, 3.5 cm in diameter. No metastatic carcinoma was found in the axillary lymph nodes.

A, mammogram, mediolateral view: Showing a diffusely infiltrating tumor (**a**) which has not formed a solid mass. There is some retraction and thickening of the skin of the breast around the nipple (**b**).

B, localized compression spot film, craniocaudal projection: Demonstration of the tumor is improved by the compression spot film in this case.

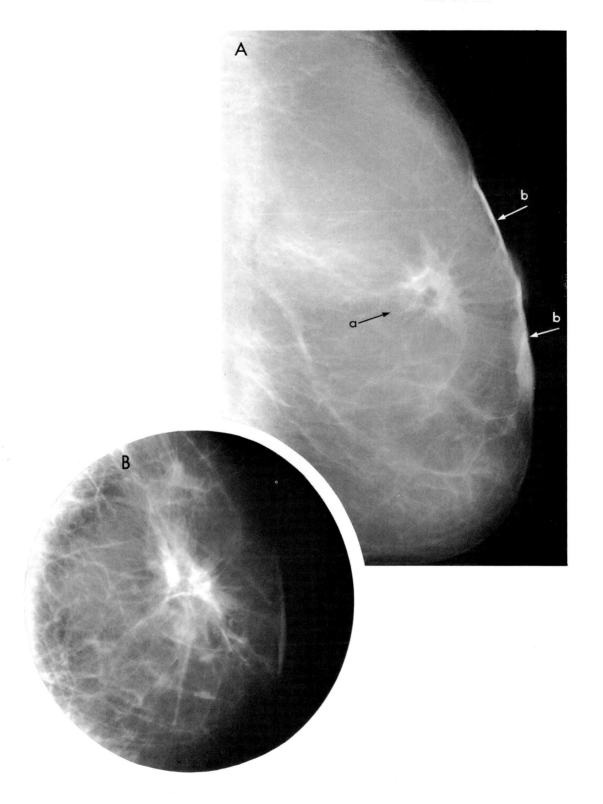

Figure 77 · Carcinoma: Invasive Pattern / 177

Figure 78.—Carcinoma with diffuse invasive pattern and no distinct mass.

A 52-year-old woman had had progressive enlargement of the right breast for several months. An ill-defined mass and unusual firmness of the breast tissue were palpated in the medial aspect of the right breast. Right radical mastectomy was performed. Pathologically, the lesion was a multi-centric grade 3 mixed comedo- and scirrhous adenocarcinoma, involving a region 6 × 5 × 4 cm of the right breast. One axillary lymph node contained metastatic tumor.

A, right breast, craniocaudal view: An ill-defined increase of density and prominent irregular breast tissue (**a**) are evident in the medial aspect of the breast. There are no specific signs of carcinoma; however, when compared with the opposite breast (**B**), there is a marked difference in architectural pattern suggesting the presence of diffuse disease.

B, left breast, craniocaudal view: Normal opposite breast shown for comparison.

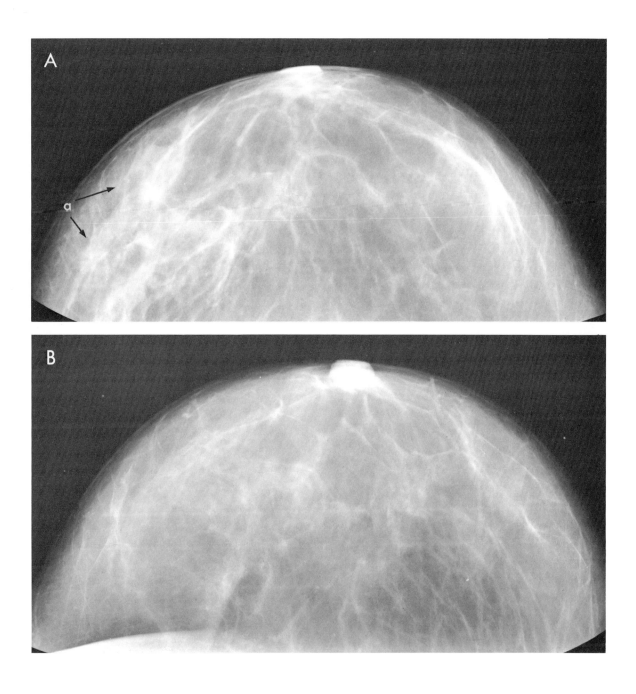

Figure 78 · Carcinoma: Diffuse Invasive Pattern / 179

Figure 79.—Carcinoma with diffuse invasive pattern involving entire breast.

A 32-year-old woman had a tender and enlarging right breast. Both breasts were nodular to palpation, but the right was firm and more nodular than the left. Clinically, she had fibrocystic disease. Right radical mastectomy was performed. Pathologically, the lesion was a diffuse grade 4 adenocarcinoma involving the greater portion of the breast. Multiple (15) lymph nodes were found to be metastatically involved.

A, right breast, mediolateral view: A diffuse increase of density is seen throughout the breast. No mass is evident. A few scattered calcifications suggestive of benign disease are present (**arrow**). The architectural pattern of the breast is abnormal when compared with the other (**B**).

B, left breast, mediolateral view: Normal breast with moderately glandular parenchyma.

Comment: This case and the preceding one (Fig. **78**) illustrate the importance of comparison of the mammograms of the two breasts. The only clue to the presence of diffuse carcinoma in these cases is the generalized increase of density and the disordered architectural pattern of one breast, which is seen when the normal and abnormal breasts are compared.

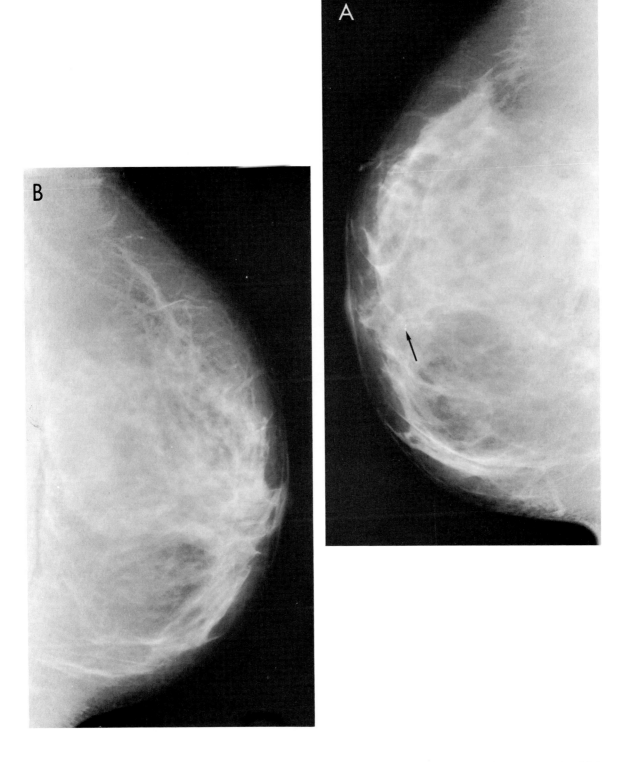

Figure 79 · Carcinoma: Diffuse Invasive Pattern / 181

Figure 80.—Subareolar carcinoma: characteristic appearance.

A 68-year-old woman had a hard mass beneath the left nipple. Radical mastectomy was performed. Pathologically, the lesion was a grade 3 subareolar scirrhous adenocarcinoma, 2.5 cm in diameter. The tumor extended along lactiferous ducts and lymphatics into the nipple.

A, entire breast, craniocaudal view.

B, enlarged localized view to show details of the tumor.

There is a typical opaque carcinomatous mass with an invasive spiculated posterior margin (**arrows**) in the subareolar area (**a**). The lesion extends to the skin; there are thickening of the skin (**b**), of the nipple and areola and slight retraction of the nipple. A small area of coarse benign calcification is present laterally in the breast (**c**).

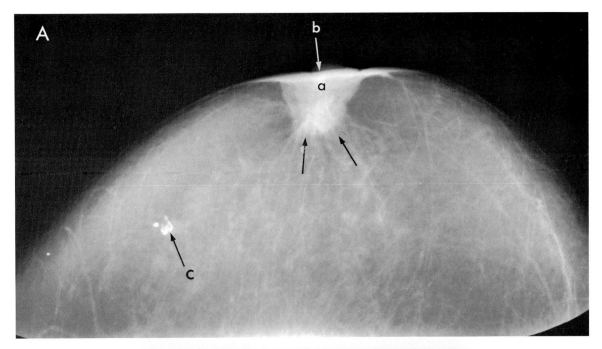

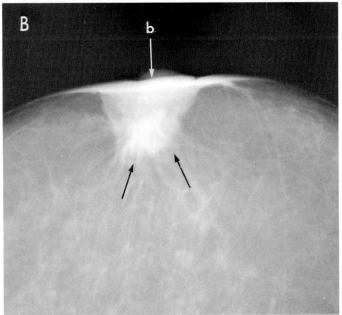

Figure 80 · Subareolar Carcinoma / 183

Figure 81.—Subareolar carcinoma associated with diffuse fibrocystic disease.

A 63-year-old woman had diffuse fibrocystic disease of many years' duration. Recently, a mass had appeared in the right breast beneath the nipple. Radical mastectomy was performed. Pathologically, the lesion was a scirrhous adenocarcinoma, 4 cm in diameter, arising beneath the nipple and areola. Diffuse fibrocystic disease of the fibrous type was found throughout the remainder of the breast.

Mammogram, craniocaudal view: The dense nodular breast has an area of greater density beneath the nipple (**arrows**). The architectural pattern of the subareolar area is abnormal, suggesting invasive tumor.

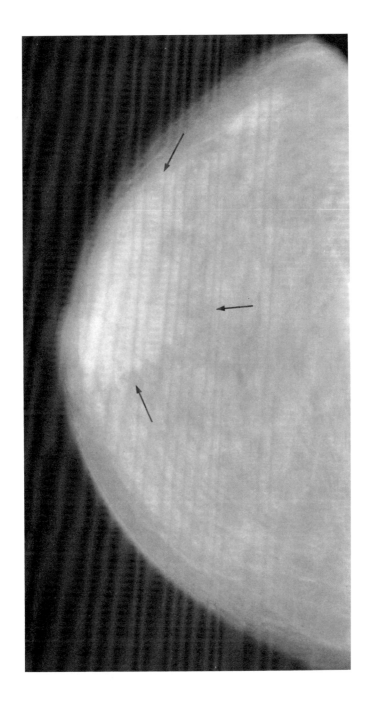

Figure 81 · Subareolar Carcinoma: With Fibrocystic Disease / 185

Figure 82.—Subareolar carcinoma: variations in mammographic appearance.

A, subareolar fibrous tissue obscures the tumor. Skin thickening and nipple retraction are present.

B, an ill-defined subareolar mass contains many tiny punctate tumor calcifications (**arrow**). There is associated nipple retraction and thickening.

C, a carcinoma (**arrows**), 2.5 cm in diameter, at some distance beneath the areola is partially obscured by subareolar fibrosis. Two tiny calcifications are present in the tumor.

D, a subareolar carcinoma, 1 cm in diameter, is completely obscured by dense subareolar fibrosis associated with comedomastitis. The only evidence of tumor is the thickening of the skin of the areola.

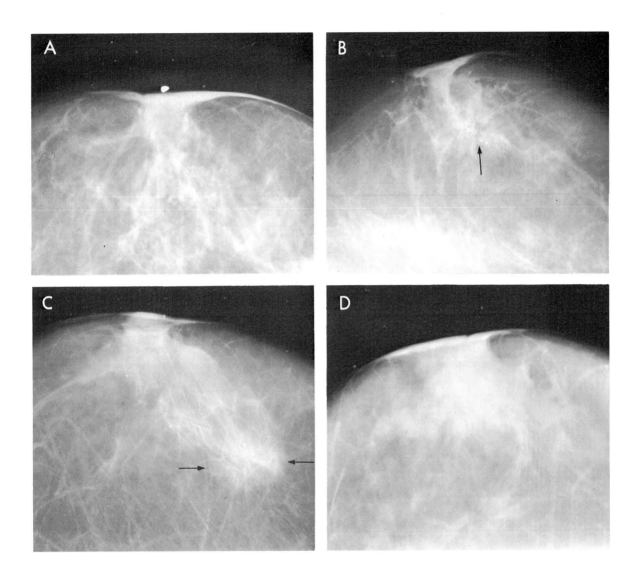

Figure 82 · Subareolar Carcinoma: Variable Appearance / 187

Figure 83.—Subareolar carcinoma obscured by ductal ectasia (comedomastitis).

A 76-year-old woman had a long history of "mastitis." There had been inversion of the nipples bilaterally for many years. Bilateral subareolar masses were palpable on physical examination. Left simple mastectomy with axillary dissection and right simple mastectomy were performed. Pathologically, the lesion in the left breast was a subareolar scirrhous carcinoma, 2 cm in diameter, with extensive comedomastitis and calcification. The axillary lymph nodes were not involved. The lesion in the right breast was comedomastitis with calcification.

A, left breast, craniocaudal view.

B, right breast, localized view of subareolar area.

Dense irregular breast parenchyma is seen beneath both nipples. Coarse calcifications typical of comedomastitis are present. Both nipples are retracted, but the change is greater in the left nipple (**a**) where the carcinoma is located than in the right, and the subareolar tissues are of greater density (**b**). A diagnosis of carcinoma can be suspected but cannot be made with certainty in the left breast, however.

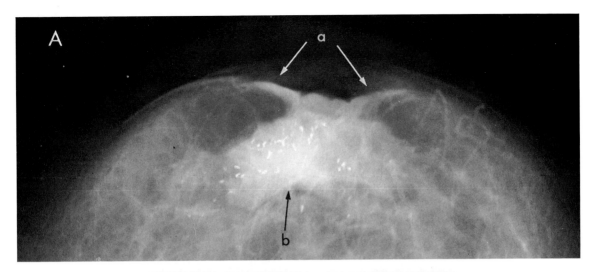

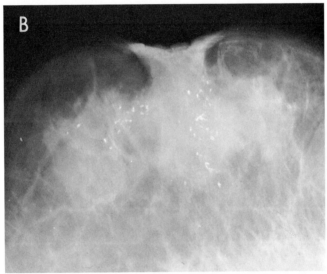

Figure 83 · Subareolar Carcinoma: With Ductal Ectasia / 189

Figure 84.—Calcification in carcinoma: characteristic features.

A 41-year-old woman had a large ill-defined mass in the upper part of the left breast. Radical mastectomy was performed. Pathologically, the lesion comprised multicentric mixed comedo-, scirrhous and papillary carcinoma, involving most of the upper half of the breast.

Mammogram, mediolateral view: Punctate calcifications (**arrows**) characteristic of carcinoma are seen throughout a large but localized area in the upper half of the breast. The calcifications are irregular in outline, variable in size (ranging down to the limits of visibility) and uncountable. The breast is moderately glandular, and the tumor mass is not well demonstrated.

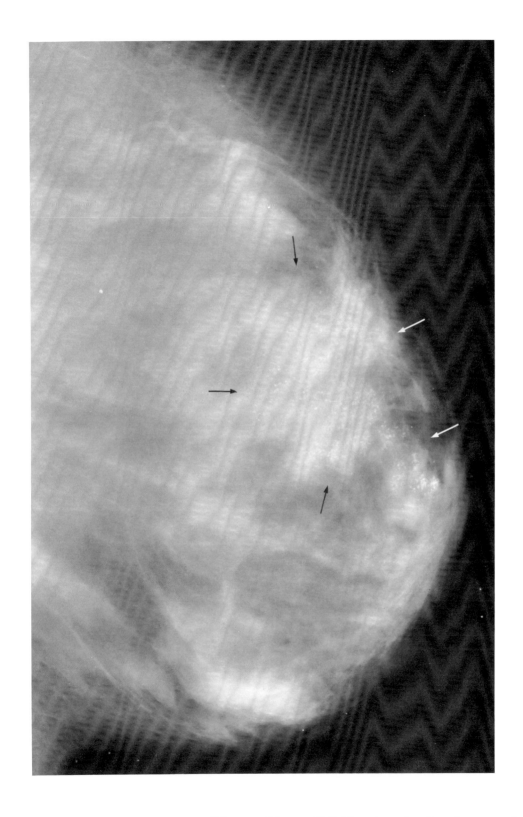

Figure 84 · Calcification in Carcinoma / 191

Figure 85.—Calcification in carcinoma: characteristic features in discrete mass.

A 65-year-old woman had a recently discovered hard mass in the upper outer quadrant of the left breast. Radical mastectomy was performed. Pathologically, the lesion comprised multicentric grade 3 mixed comedo- and scirrhous adenocarcinoma in multiple nodules ranging up to 2.5 cm in diameter. Axillary lymph nodes were free from tumor.

A, entire breast, mediolateral view.

B, enlarged segment of mammogram to show details of calcification.

A poorly defined, multinodular tumor is present in the upper portion of the breast. Innumerable calcific flecks are present in and around the mass (**a**). The sizes of the calcifications vary widely and most are angular in outline, although the largest appear somewhat rounded. A separate tiny collection of calcifications is present a few centimeters anterior to the main mass in a separate tiny nodule of tumor (**b**).

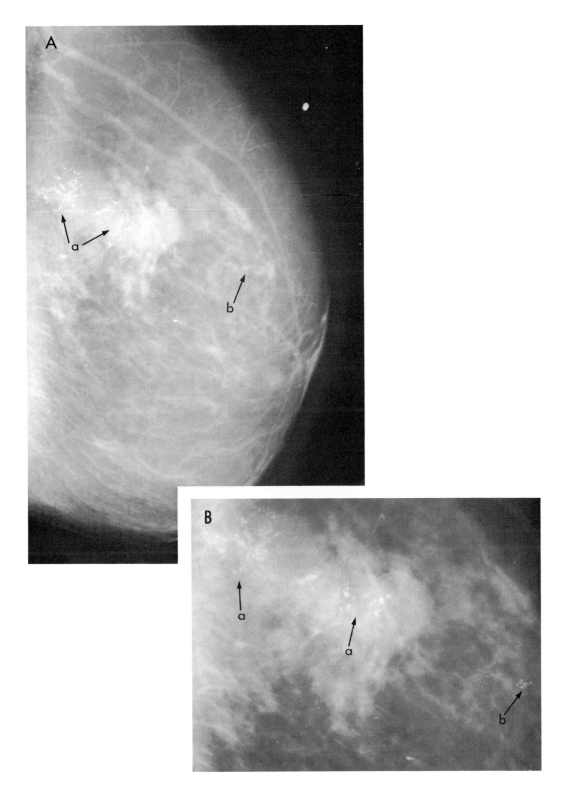

Figure 85 · Calcification in Carcinoma / 193

Figure 86.—Calcification in carcinoma: variations in pattern.

A, mammogram: A well-formed scirrhous carcinoma has calcifications localized in its center (**arrow**).

B, enlarged segment of mammogram to show details of calcification: Innumerable punctate calcifications (**arrows**) of various sizes and shapes in and around a large invasive carcinoma of a mixed scirrhous, lobular and comedo type.

C, craniocaudal view: "Lacelike" calcification (**arrows**) in poorly defined scirrhous carcinoma. The calcification appears in three separate nodules representing different deposits of tumor.

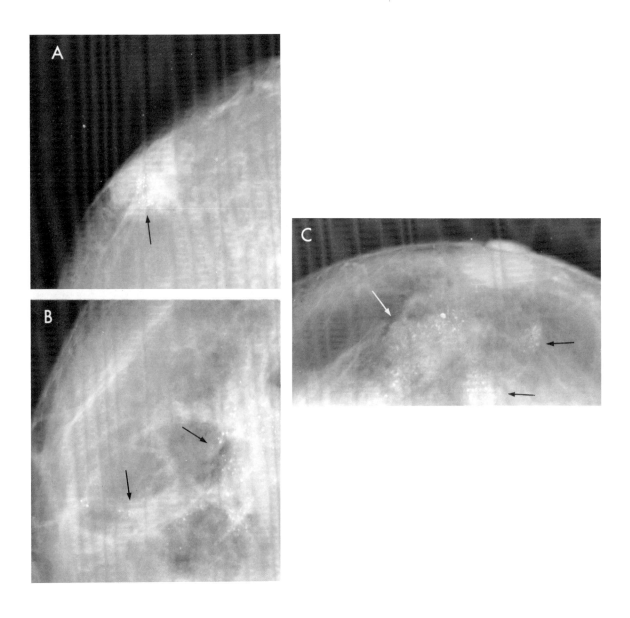

Figure 86 · Calcification in Carcinoma: Variable Patterns / 195

Figure 87.—Calcification in carcinoma: linear distribution along ducts.

A 66-year-old woman had multiple ill-defined nodules in the right breast and several large palpable axillary lymph nodes. Radical mastectomy was performed. Pathologically, multicentric nodules of grade 4 scirrhous adenocarcinoma, varying from 0.2 to 3 cm in diameter, were scattered throughout the breast. Calcification was present in several carcinoma-filled ducts. Multiple axillary nodes were involved by metastatic carcinoma.

Mammogram, enlarged segment of mediolateral view: The deposits of tumor are difficult to identify, although an irregular density is seen in the upper part of the breast (**a**). Typical punctate tumor calcifications (**b**) are located beneath the nipple and extend in a linear fashion along a dilated duct to the mass in the upper part of the breast.

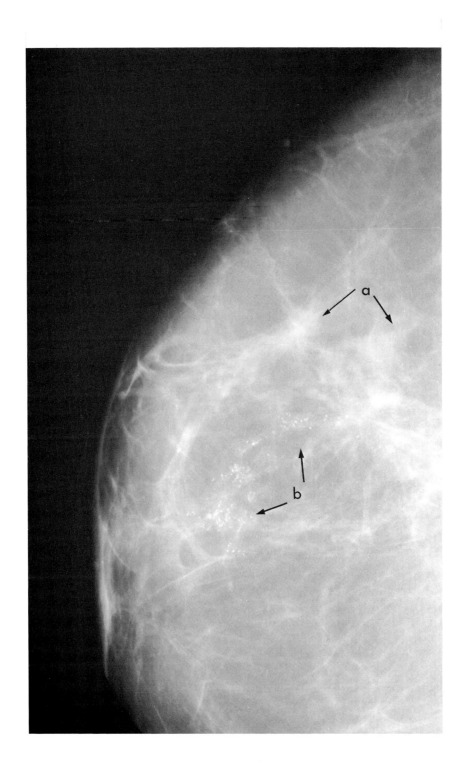

Figure 87 · Calcification in Carcinoma: Linear Distribution / 197

Figure 88.—Calcification in carcinoma: coarse type.

A, a single coarse rounded calcification (**arrow**) is associated with a typical infiltrating scirrhous carcinoma.

B, two coarse rounded calcifications (**arrow**) that appear to be homogeneous in density are present in an irregular scirrhous carcinoma.

C, several coarse irregular but very dense calcifications (**a**) are in a small (2 cm) scirrhous carcinoma. Linear arterial calcification (**b**) overlies the lower margin of the tumor.

Comment: Coarse calcifications of the types illustrated here are frequently found in carcinoma. These calcifications are indistinguishable from calcifications found in benign disease and are of little value in differential diagnosis.

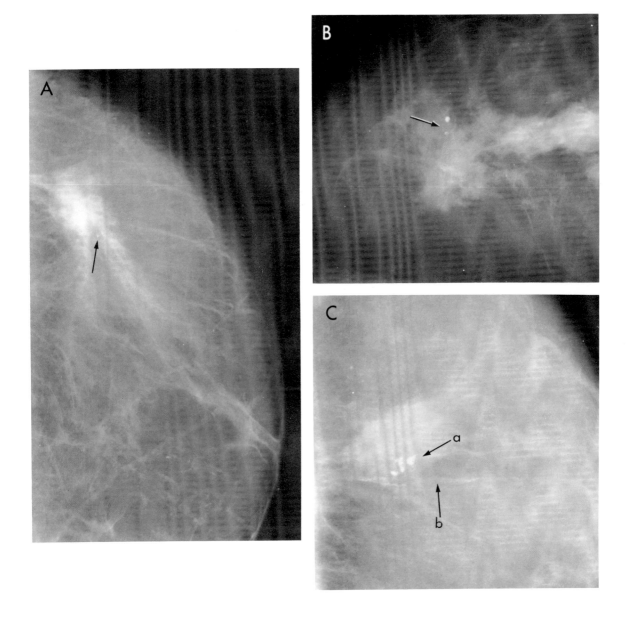

Figure 88 · Calcification in Carcnoma: Coarse Type / 199

Figure 89.—Calcification in carcinoma: only evidence of tumor in a dense breast.

A 51-year-old woman had a long history of fibrocystic disease. The breasts were nodular, but no dominant, clinically suspect mass was present. Excisional biopsy was performed on the basis of the mammographic report of probable carcinoma, and carcinoma was found in the specimen. Radical mastectomy was performed. Pathologically, the lesion was a grade 3 scirrhous adenocarcinoma, 1.5 cm in diameter, containing calcification. Three axillary lymph nodes were involved by metastatic tumor.

Mammogram, enlargement of craniocaudal view to illustrate calcification: The breast is dense throughout due to presence of fibrocystic disease of the fibrous type. A small localized area of punctate calcification (**arrow**) typical of carcinoma is seen in the upper part of the breast. No associated mass can be seen.

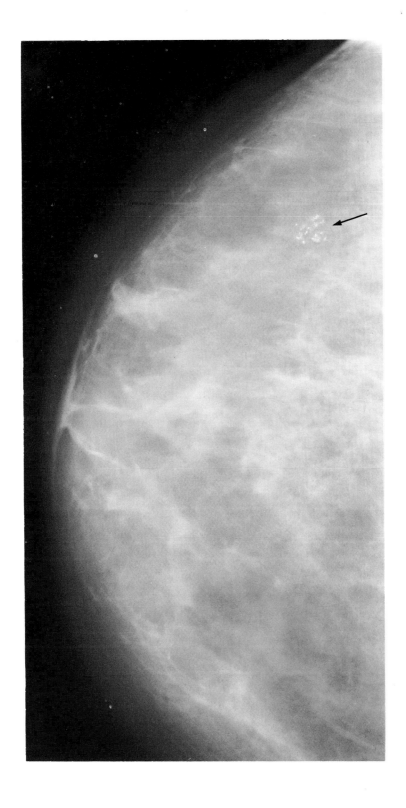

Figure 89 · Calcification in Carcinoma / 201

Figure 90.—Calcification in carcinoma: only evidence of tumor associated with a palpable benign nodule.

A 63-year-old woman had a palpable, clinically benign nodule in the lateral portion of the breast. Excisional biopsy of the palpable mass revealed fibrocystic disease, but a repeat biopsy on the basis of the mammographic report of carcinoma revealed underlying tumor. Radical mastectomy was performed. Pathologically, the lesion was a grade 4 adenocarcinoma, 2 cm in diameter. Axillary lymph nodes were free from tumor.

Segment of mammogram enlarged to show details of the calcification: The benign palpable cyst (**a**) is seen lying in front of a localized area of typical punctate tumor calcification (**b**). No mass can be identified in association with the calcification.

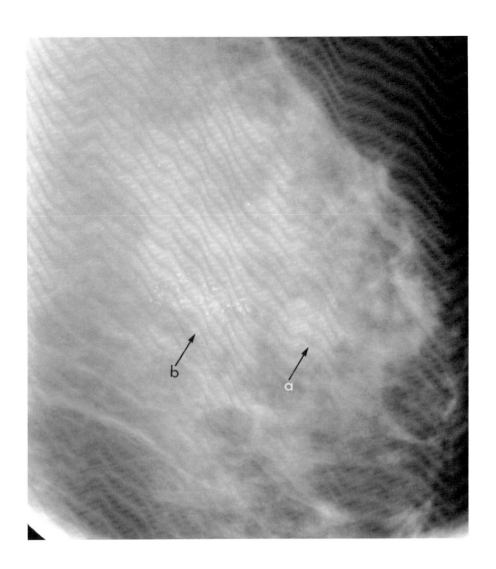

Figure 90 · Calcification in Carcinoma / 203

Figure 91.—Calcification in benign disease simulating malignant type of calcification.

A, enlarged segment of mammogram: Innumerable calcifications (**arrows**) of various sizes are present in the central part of the breast of a 66-year-old woman. Most are irregular in outline, suggesting carcinoma. Biopsy, on the basis of the mammographic report of carcinoma, revealed diffuse fibrocystic disease with calcifications in and around dilated ducts.

B, segment of mammogram: A localized area of calcification (**arrows**) is present in the central portion of the breast of a 51-year-old woman. The calcifications are punctate, irregular in outline and variable in size. Biopsy, on the basis of the mammographic report of probable carcinoma, revealed localized fibrocystic disease with foci of intraductal calcification.

C, segment of mammogram: A small collection of calcifications (**arrow**) is present in the moderately dense breast of a 57-year-old woman. The calcifications are irregular in outline and variable in size. Biopsy, on the basis of the mammographic diagnosis of possible carcinoma, revealed a localized area of "mastitis" with foci of calcification in the ducts.

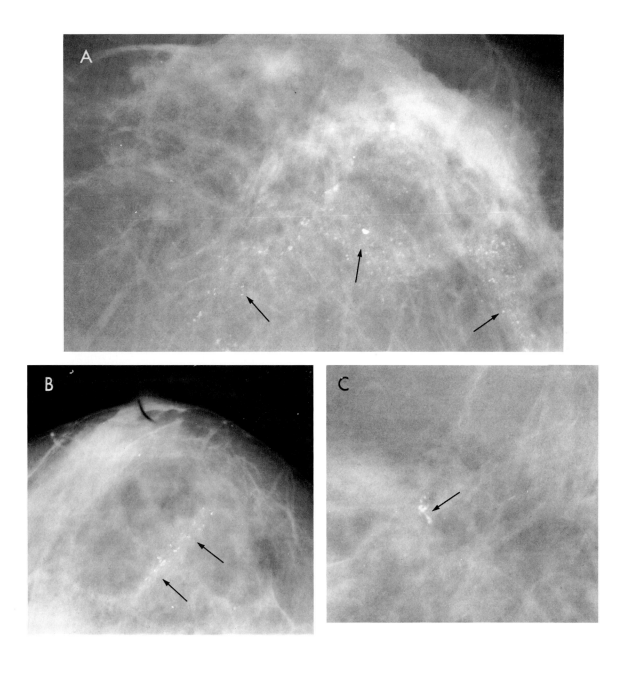

Figure 91 · Calcification in Benign Disease: Differentiation / 205

Figure 92.—Carcinoma with localized skin thickening.

A 61-year-old woman had a mass above the right areola in the mid-portion of the breast. There was flattening of the skin over the tumor which clinically was diagnosed as carcinoma. Radical mastectomy was performed. Pathologically, the lesion was a scirrhous adenocarcinoma, 2.5 cm in diameter, with overlying thickening of the skin.

Enlarged portion of mammogram, mediolateral view: A typical stellate carcinoma (**a**) is located well below the skin. The skin overlying the tumor is thickened and flattened (**b**). Two prominent vessels (**c**) which may be dilated lymphatics are present just beneath the segment of thickened skin.

Comment: Often skin thickening can be detected on the mammogram weeks or months before it is apparent clinically. In some instances, especially in dense breasts, it is the only radiographic evidence of carcinoma.

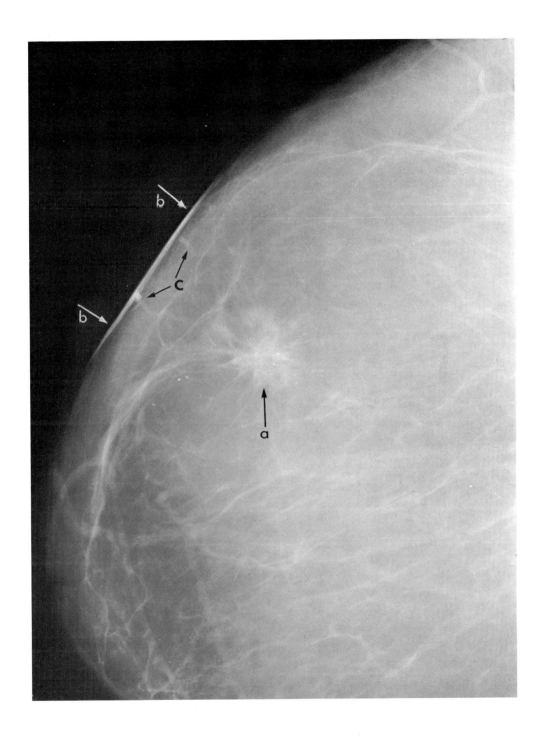

Figure 92 · Carcinoma: Localized Skin Thickening / 207

Figure 93.—Carcinoma with diffuse skin thickening.

A 60-year-old woman had a large mass involving the central portion of one breast. The skin was thickened over the entire breast, but the thickening was greatest in the lower half. Clinically, the lesion represented carcinoma. Radical mastectomy was performed. Pathologically, the specimen contained a diffuse grade 4 adenocarcinoma involving the greater portion of the breast. Multiple axillary lymph nodes were involved by metastatic carcinoma.

Mammogram, mediolateral view: There is a diffuse increase of density throughout the breast with skin thickening over the entire breast. An ill-defined mass (**a**) is present in the center of the breast. The thickening of the skin (**b**) is greater around the nipple and in the lower portion of the breast than elsewhere. The normal architectural pattern of the breast is destroyed and the subcutaneous fat line partially obliterated. Dilated lymphatics (**c**) are present just deep to the skin.

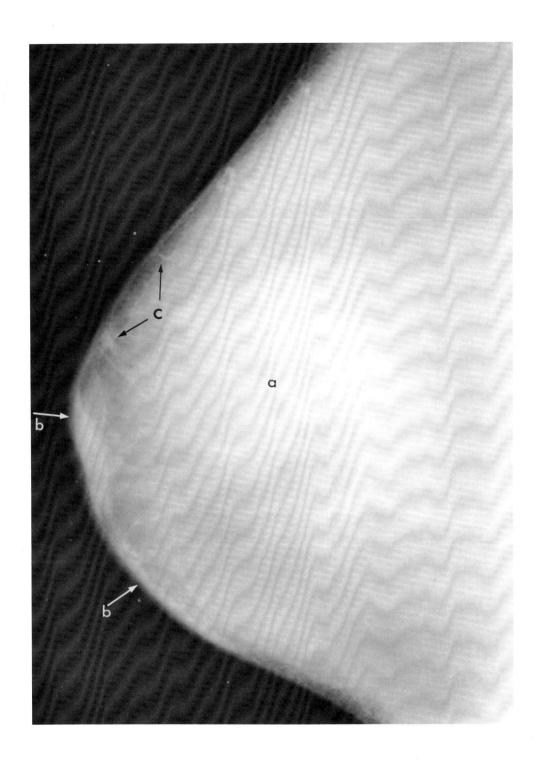

Figure 93 · Carcinoma: Diffuse Skin Thickening / 209

Figure 94.—Carcinoma in a dense breast with diffuse skin thickening.

A 47-year-old woman with known fibrocystic disease had recent onset of pain in the left breast with rapid enlargement of the breast. The clinical diagnosis was carcinoma. Radical mastectomy was performed. Pathologically, extensive grade 4 scirrhous adenocarcinoma was found in the central portion of the breast beneath the nipple. There was thickening of the skin with clumps of cancer cells in the lymphatics of the skin.

Mammogram, craniocaudal view: Diffuse skin thickening is greatest in the region of the areola (**a**). The primary tumor (**b**), which is located in a subareolar position, is difficult to see. The subcutaneous fat line (**c**) is obliterated. The architectural pattern of the breast, especially in its central portion, is disrupted.

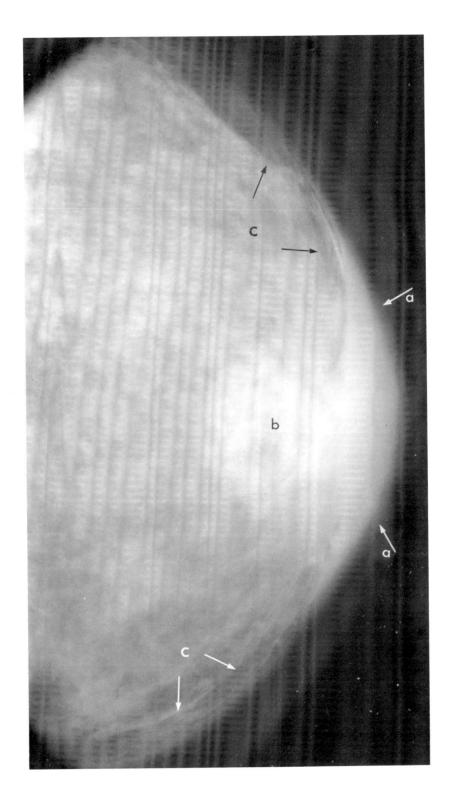

Figure 94 · Carcinoma: Diffuse Skin Thickening / 211

Figure 95.—Inflammatory carcinoma.

A 50-year-old woman had recent onset of swelling, pain and inflammation of the left breast. Clinically, the lesion was inflammatory carcinoma with classic peau d'orange appearance of the skin. Biopsy was performed, followed by irradiation therapy. Pathologically, there was diffuse grade 4 scirrhous adenocarcinoma with involvement of the skin and the dermal lymphatics.

A, left breast, craniocaudal view: The skin of the breast (**arrows**) is diffusely thickened, but the thickening is greatest in the lateral half. The left breast is much more dense than the right (see **B**). No other evidence of carcinoma is seen.

B, right breast, craniocaudal view: Normal breast, shown for comparison.

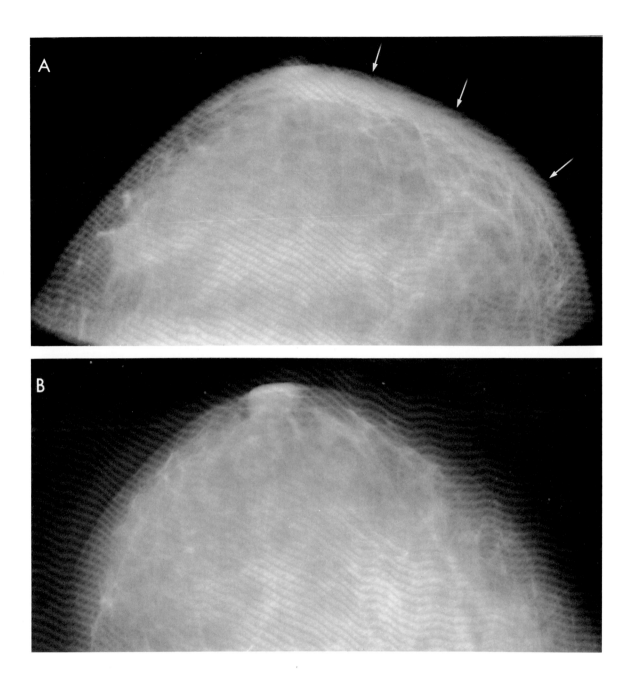

Figure 95 · Inflammatory Carcinoma / 213

Figure 96.—Carcinoma with increased vascularity.

A 76-year-old woman had a nodular lesion in the upper outer quadrant of the left breast. Radical mastectomy was performed. Pathologically, the lesion was grade 4 scirrhous adenocarcinoma, 2.5 cm in diameter. Multiple axillary lymph nodes were involved by metastatic carcinoma.

A, left breast, craniocaudal view: An ill-defined spiculated mass (**a**) is in the upper outer quadrant. The veins (**b**) are more than twice as wide in this breast as they are in the right breast (see **B**), indicating increased blood flow associated with the tumor.

B, right breast, craniocaudal view: Normal opposite breast, shown for comparison, has some residual fibrotic parenchyma throughout (**x**), but the veins (**arrows**) are of normal size.

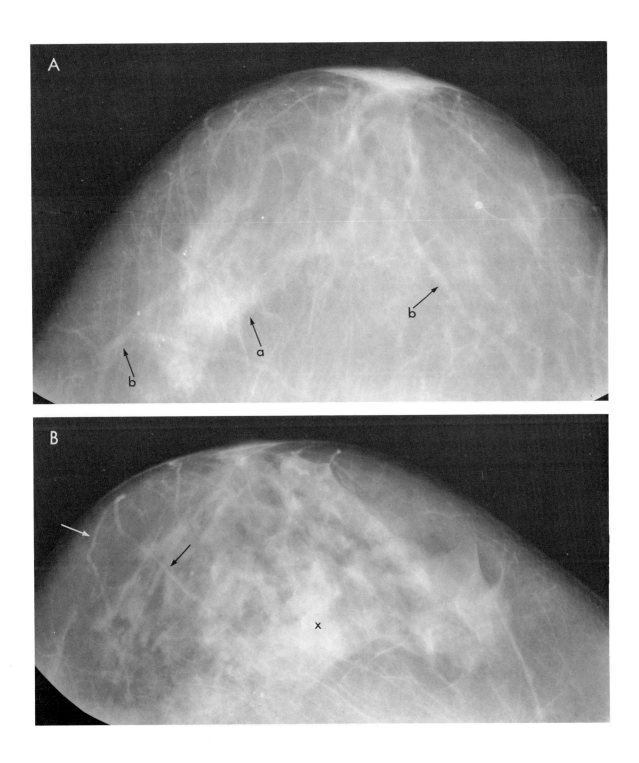

Figure 96 · Carcinoma: With Increased Vascularity / 215

Figure 97.—Increased vascularity localized to the region of a carcinoma.

A 71-year-old woman had a large mass in the upper outer quadrant of the left breast. Clinically, the lesion was carcinoma. Radical mastectomy was performed. Pathologically, there was a grade 4 scirrhous adenocarcinoma, 4 cm in diameter. Axillary lypmh nodes were free from tumor.

Enlarged segment of a localized area in the upper part of the breast: There is a large spiculated tumor (**a**) with numerous large veins (**b**) radiating from it. There was no evidence of increased vascularity in other parts of the breast.

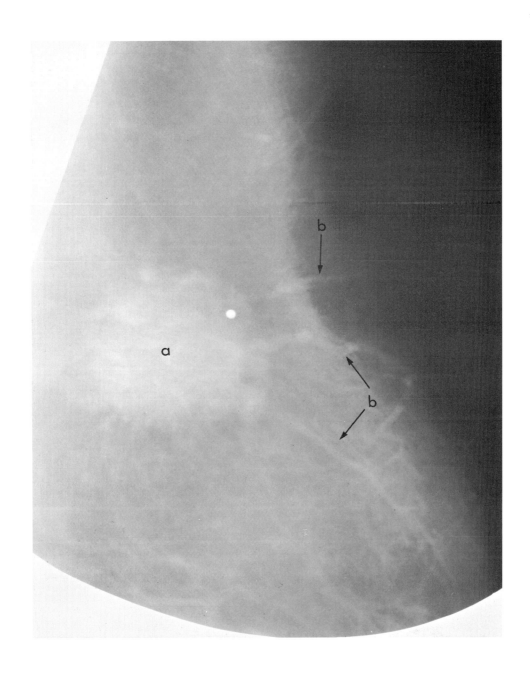

Figure 97 · Carcinoma: With Increased Vascularity / 217

Figure 98.—Carcinoma undetected but for increased vascularity.

A 77-year-old woman had "thickening" but no definite mass in the tail of the right breast. Biopsy was made on the basis of mammographic diagnosis of carcinoma. Radical mastectomy was performed. Pathologically, there was a grade 4 scirrhous adenocarcinoma, 2 cm in diameter, high in the upper outer quadrant. Many axillary lymph nodes were involved metastatically.

A, mammogram, mediolateral view: There is a marked increase in the size of the veins (**arrows**) of the breast. No mass is seen, but the venous enlargement suggested the need for further views.

B, localized compression spot view (enlarged) of the axillary extension of the breast: A typical circumscribed carcinoma (**a**) with associated increased vascularity (**b**) is seen.

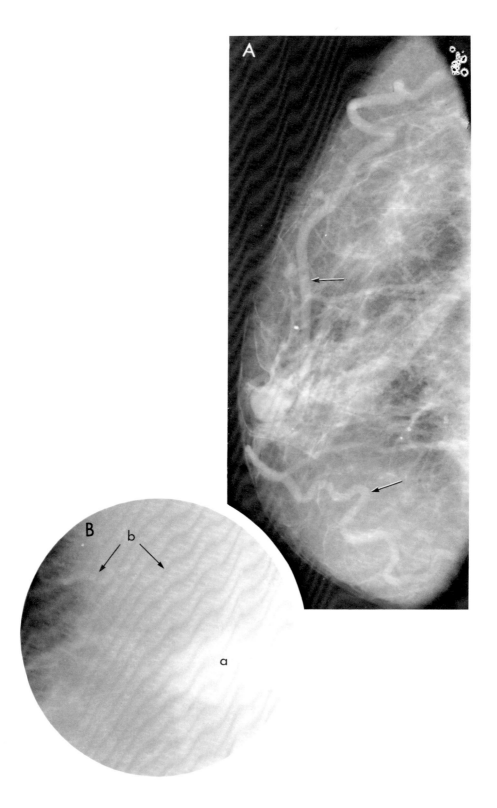

Figure 98 · Carcinoma: With Increased Vascularity / 219

Figure 99.—Carcinoma with nipple retraction.

A 61-year-old woman had a hard mass beneath the right nipple, which was thickened and retracted. Clinically, the lesion was carcinoma. Radical mastectomy was performed. Pathologically, the lesion was a grade 3 scirrhous adenocarcinoma, 2 cm in diameter, with foci of grade 2 intraductal carcinoma. Axillary lymph nodes were not involved.

A, right breast, craniocaudal view: A typical circumscribed carcinoma (**a**) is present beneath the nipple. The nipple (**b**) is retracted, and the skin of the nipple and areola is thickened. Increased vascularity (**c**) is apparent.

B, left breast, craniocaudal view: Normal opposite breast shown for comparison.

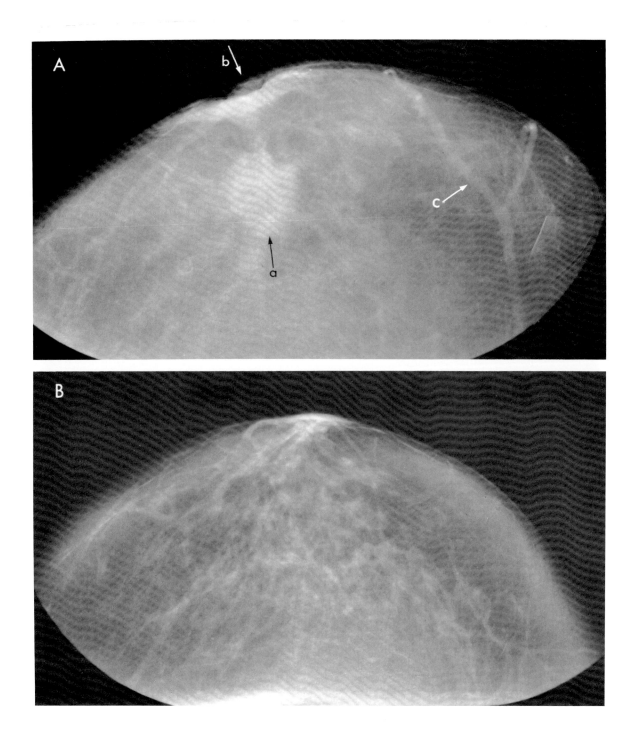

Figure 99 · Carcinoma: With Nipple Retraction / 221

Figure 100.—Nipple retraction: congenital and malignant.

A 72-year-old woman had had retraction of the nipples of both breasts since adolescence. A recent increase of the retraction on the left was associated with the development of a large palpable mass in the midportion of the breast. Radical mastectomy was performed. Pathologically, the lesion in the left breast was a diffuse grade 4 adenocarcinoma involving the central portion of the breast and extending into the nipple.

A, left breast, craniocaudal view: There is a large carcinoma (**a**) in the subareolar position with nipple retraction (**b**) and skin thickening.

B, portion of right breast, mediolateral view: There is congenital inversion of the nipple (**arrow**). Note that no thickening of the skin of the nipple or areola is present.

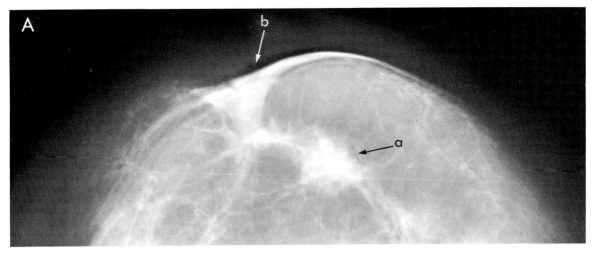

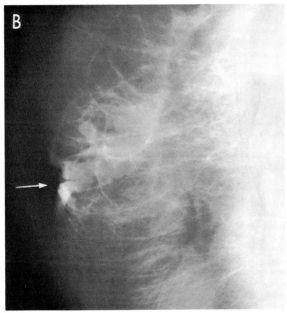

Figure 100 · Nipple Retraction: Congenital and Malignant / 223

Figure 101.—Carcinoma with skin retraction.

A 90-year-old woman had had a large mass in the left breast for more than a year. The skin was retracted and deformed over the tumor. Simple mastectomy was performed, with removal of axillary nodes (palliative). Pathologically, the lesion was a grade 4 infiltrating ductal carcinoma, 6 cm in diameter, with metastasis to many axillary lymph nodes. The tumor extended to the skin.

Mammogram, craniocaudal view: The skin (**a**) over the tumor (**b**) is thickened and retracted. The tumor is multinodular and contains a single coarse calcification.

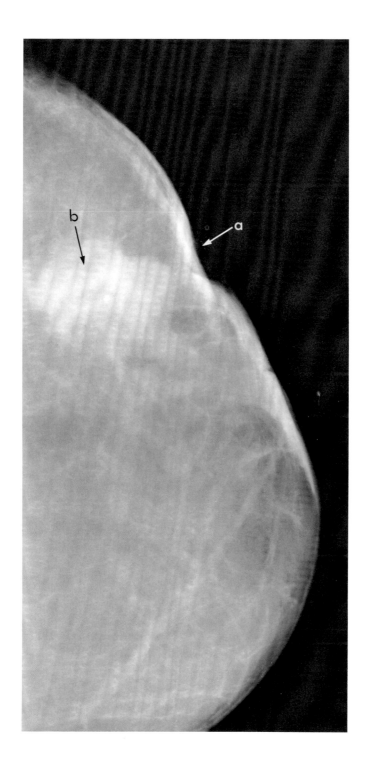

Figure 101 · Carcinoma: With Skin Retraction / 225

Figure 102.—Carcinoma with ulceration.

A, craniocaudal view: A huge ulcerated carcinoma occupies the central portion of the breast. The skin of the entire breast is thickened. The ulcerated area (**arrows**) is large in diameter but shallow.

B, mammogram, portion of mediolateral view: An ulcerated carcinoma is located in the lower part of the breast. The lesion invades the chest wall posteriorly (**a**) and is deeply ulcerated (**b**) in its center.

C, mammogram, portion of mediolateral view: A large carcinoma (**a**) of the upper portion of the breast has invaded the skin. There are deformity and thickening of the skin and a small area of ulceration (**b**) at the upper margin of the lesion.

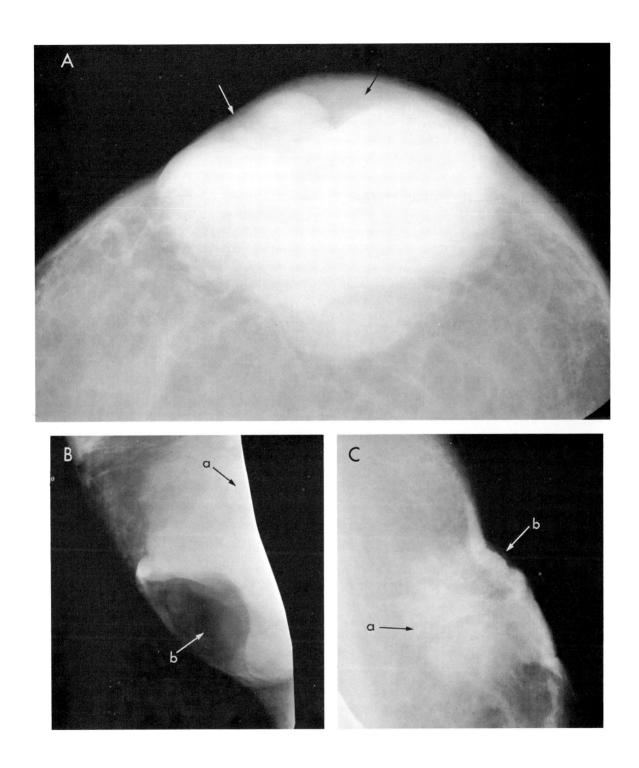

Figure 102 · Carcinoma: With Ulceration / 227

Figure 103.—Carcinoma invading the chest wall.

A, mammogram, mediolateral view: A large carcinoma in the upper part of the breast extends to, but not through, the retromammary space (**arrows**). Compare with **B.**

B, mammogram, mediolateral view: A large carcinoma in the lower part of the breast has invaded the anterior chest wall and obliterated the retromammary space (**arrows**).

Figure 103, **B,** courtesy of Dr. Robert L. Scanlan, Los Angeles.

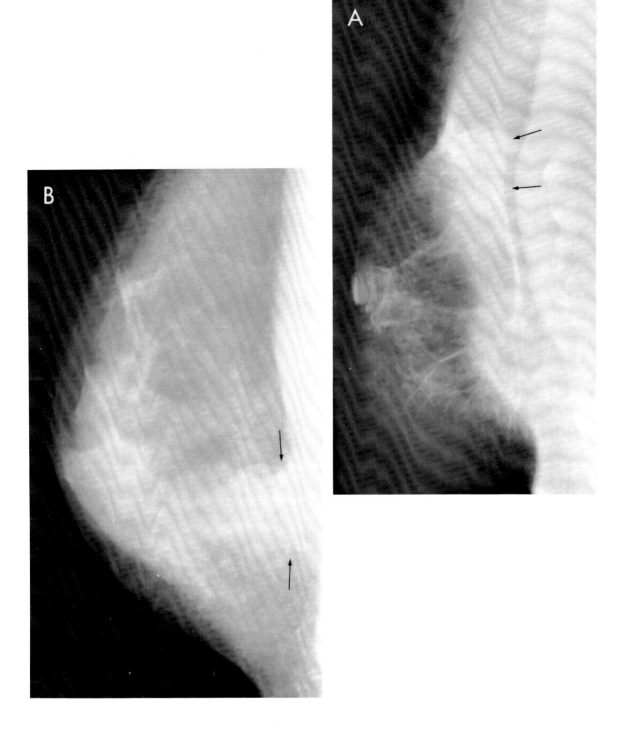

Figure 103 · Carcinoma: Invading Chest Wall / 229

Figure 104.—Enlargement of axillary lymph nodes from metastatic carcinoma.

Axillary view: Large axillary lymph node (**arrows**) contains metastatic carcinoma from a primary lesion in the breast on the same side. (See also Figure **105.**)

Figure 104, courtesy of Dr. Robert L. Scanlan, Los Angeles.

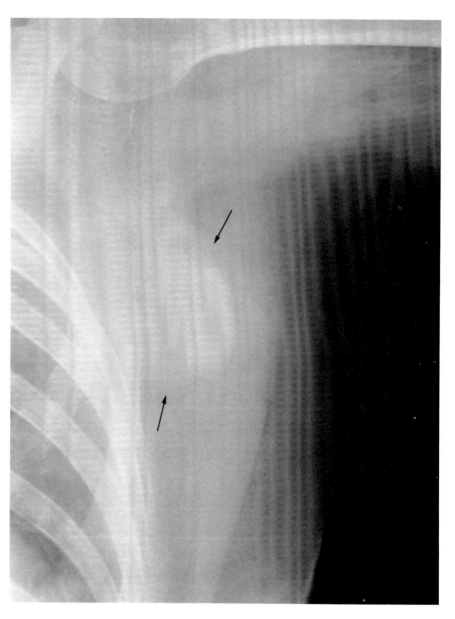

Figure 105.—Enlargement of axillary lymph nodes from metastatic carcinoma.

Axillary view: Multiple enlarged axillary lymph nodes (**arrows**) contain metastatic carcinoma from a primary lesion on the same side. The primary could not be seen on the mammogram because of dense overlying breast parenchyma. No radiographic features distinguish these enlarged nodes from nodes enlarged by inflammation or lymphoma.

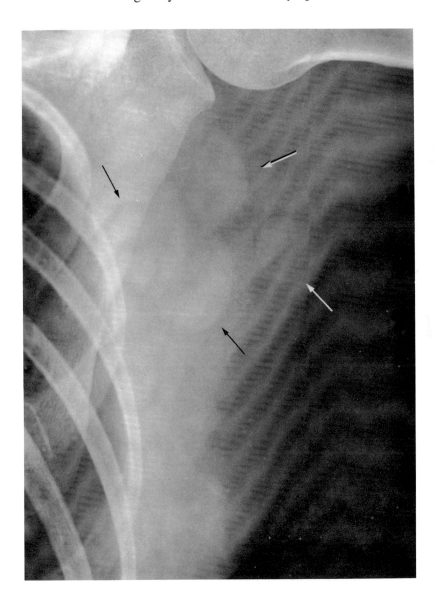

Figure 105 · Axillary Lymph Nodes / 231

Figure 106.—Calcification in metastases to axillary lymph nodes.

A, axillary view: There are calcifications (**arrows**) in deposits of metastatic carcinoma from a primary lesion in the breast. The primary was a heavily calcified carcinoma of the intraductal (comedo) type.

B, radiograph (moderately enlarged) of one of the lymph nodes containing calcified metastatic carcinoma.

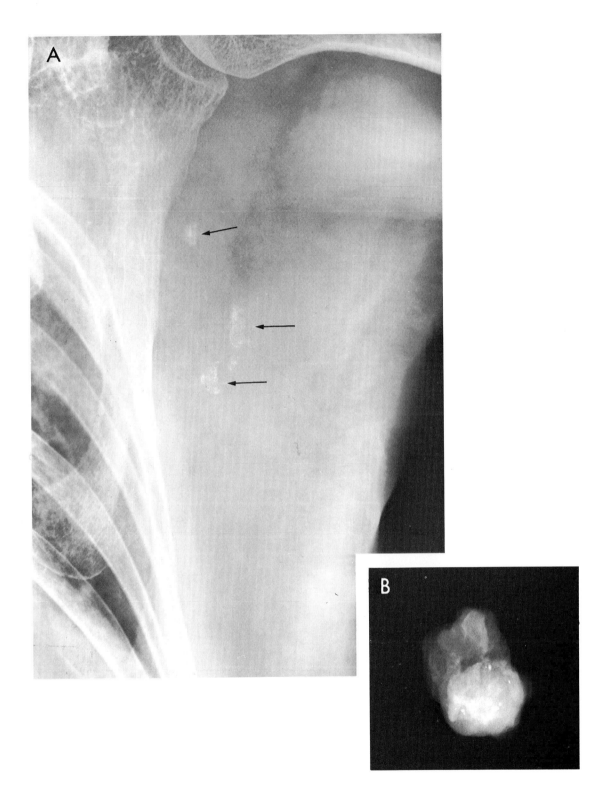

Figure 106 · Axillary Lymph Nodes / 233

Figure 107.—Noninvasive (in situ) comedocarcinoma: calcified pattern.

A 71-year-old woman had a large ill-defined mass in the upper portion of the left breast. Mastectomy was performed. Pathologically, the lesion was an in situ intraductal (comedo) carcinoma involving the ducts of the entire upper portion of the breast. The tumor was extensively calcified.

Mammogram, craniocaudal view: No tumor mass is seen. Arborizing calcific plugs (**a**) outline the mammary ducts. Typical fine punctate tumor calcifications (**b**) appear at the periphery of the larger ducts, and similar calcifications are present at a distance from the main body of the lesion.

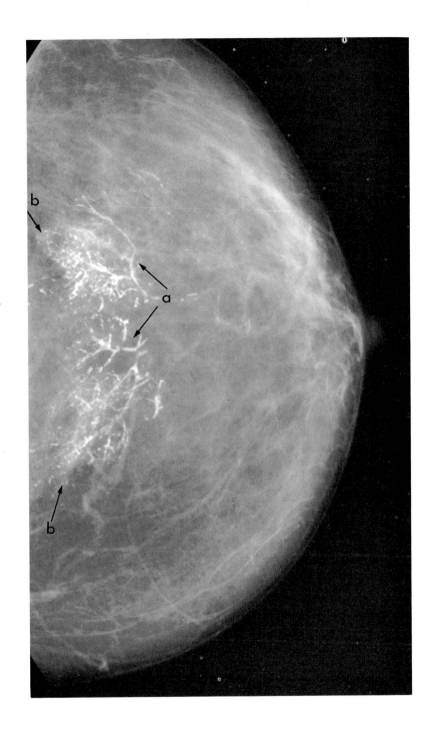

Figure 107 · Noninvasive Comedocarcinoma / 235

Figure 108.—Noninvasive (in situ) comedocarcinoma: uncalcified pattern.

A 54-year-old woman had a history of fibrocystic disease of both breasts. There was serous discharge from the left nipple and an ill-defined nodular mass in the midportion of the left breast. Left radical mastectomy was performed. Pathologically, the lesion was a multicentric grade 2 intraductal (comedo) carcinoma involving a region 7 cm in diameter. No invasion was found on multiple sections. There was associated marked fibrocystic disease with intraductal epithelial hyperplasia.

A, left breast, craniocaudal view: Dense nodular tissue is present in the central portion of the breast. This breast is more dense than its mate, but no radiographic abnormality suggesting carcinoma is seen. The appearance suggests extensive fibrocystic disease.

B, right breast, craniocaudal view: Fibrocystic changes in the central portion of this breast are shown for comparison with the opposite breast.

Comment: In the absence of calcification, the presence of in situ carcinoma can seldom be suspected from the mammogram.

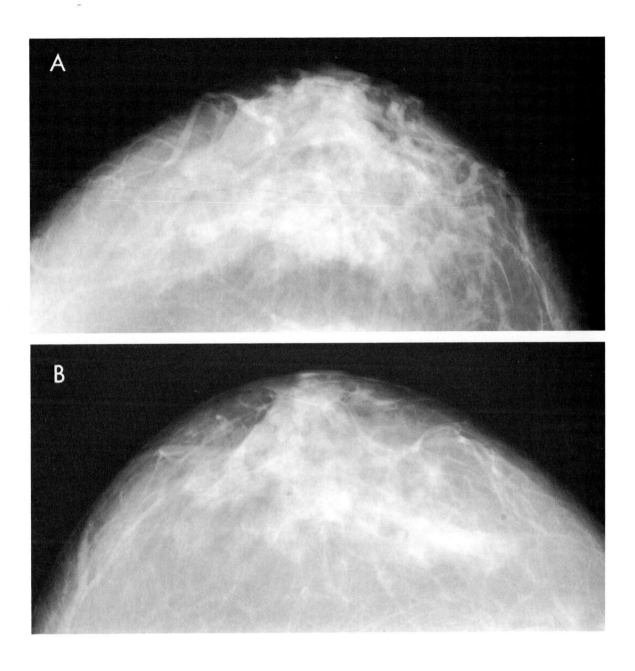

Figure 108 · Noninvasive Comedocarcinoma / 237

Figure 109.—Infiltrating comedocarcinoma in a dense breast with calcification.

A 47-year-old woman had a serosanguineous discharge from the left nipple and an ill-defined mass in the central portion of the breast. Radical mastectomy was performed. Pathologically, the lesion was an infiltrating grade 3 comedocarcinoma, 2.5 cm in diameter, with extension along the ducts toward the nipple. Axillary lymph nodes were not involved.

A, entire breast, craniocaudal view: The breast is dense and nodular due to the presence of large amounts of opaque glandular tissue. No definite mass is seen. A collection of tiny calcifications (**arrows**), typical of carcinoma, is seen beneath the nipple. These appear to extend along ducts in a linear fashion toward the nipple.

B, enlarged segment of mammogram to show details of the calcific deposits (**arrows**).

Comment: In dense breasts, calcification is often the only radiographic evidence of carcinoma.

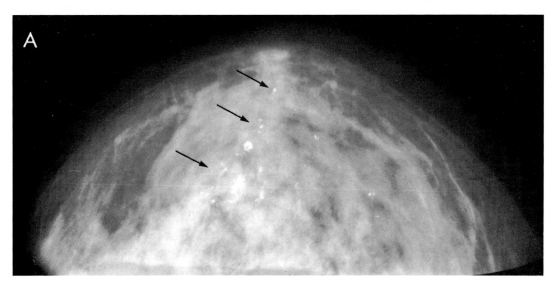

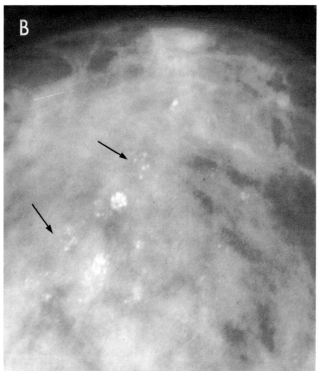

Figure 109 · Infiltrating Comedocarcinoma: Calcification / 239

Figure 110.—Infiltrating comedocarcinoma in a fatty breast.

An 83-year-old woman had a clinically indeterminate, recently discovered mass in the right breast. Simple mastectomy was performed. Pathologically, the lesion was a multicentric infiltrative grade 2 comedocarcinoma with some associated fibrosis (scirrhous reaction) in a zone about 5 cm in diameter. The individual foci measured up to 1.5 cm in diameter. The tumor extended along the ducts to the nipple.

A, entire breast, craniocaudal view: The breast is of the fatty type. Multiple small nodular densities (**arrows**) which are somewhat irregular in outline are seen in the medial half of the breast. A few tiny flecks of calcium are seen in the ducts in and beneath the nipple.

B, enlarged segment of mammogram to show calcifications in the ducts of the nipple (**arrow**).

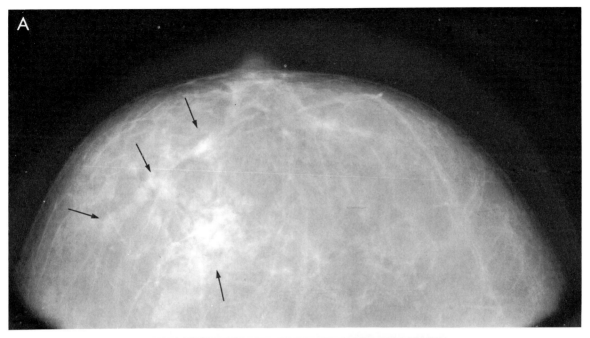

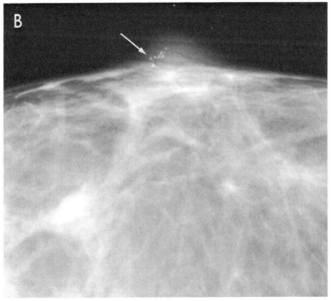

Figure 110 · Infiltrating Comedocarcinoma / 241

Figure 111.—Infiltrating comedocarcinoma: uncalcified type.

A 41-year-old woman had a discrete mass in the lower part of the right breast. She had had no previous breast complaints. Radical mastectomy was performed. Pathologically, the lesion was an infiltrating grade 3 comedocarcinoma, 3 cm in diameter. Axillary lymph nodes were free from tumor.

Mammogram, mediolateral view: The breast is dense due to the presence of large amounts of glandular tissue. The lesion in the lower portion of the breast (**arrows**) is poorly seen. (A lead shot marks the palpable nodule.) No radiographic features which would differentiate between a benign and a malignant lesion are seen in this case.

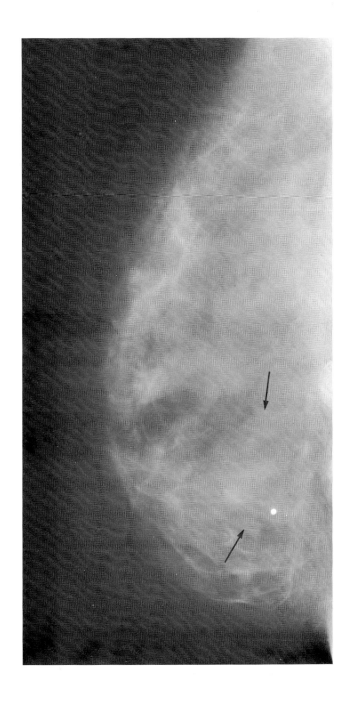

Figure 111 · Infiltrating Comedocarcinoma: Uncalcified Type / 243

Figure 112.—Infiltrating comedocarcinoma: variations in radiographic appearance.

A, discrete lesion: Part of the margin of this well-defined tumor is smooth and round (**a**) while part is infiltrative (**b**). Typical tumor calcifications are present.

B, tumor calcifications (**arrows**) arranged in a linear pattern along ducts: These provide the only evidence of a primary infiltrating comedocarcinoma with distant metastasis. No lesion was palpable in this breast, and the patient had mammography as part of the search for the primary tumor.

C, irregular, ill-defined tumor (**arrows**) in a fatty-type breast: Multiple tiny calcifications are present, and there is localized skin thickening over the lesion. Pathologically, the lesion was an infiltrative grade 3 comedocarcinoma with axillary lymph node metastasis.

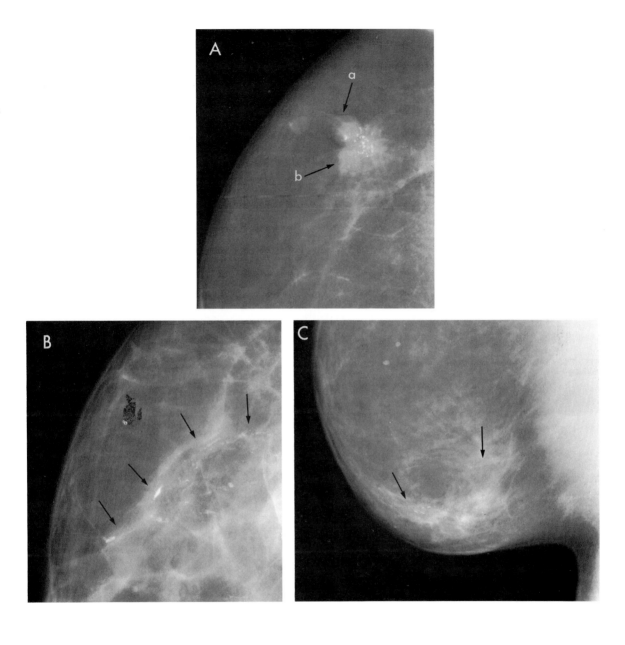

Figure 112 · Infiltrating Comedocarcinoma / 245

Figure 113.—Noninfiltrating (in situ) papillary carcinoma.

A 70-year-old woman had a mass in the lower portion of the right breast. Incisional biopsy and simple mastectomy were performed. Pathologically, the lesion was a multicentric noninfiltrating papillary intraductal carcinoma involving much of the breast.

Mammogram, craniocaudal view: The palpable portion of the lesion forms a multilobular benign-appearing mass (**a**). However, scattered punctate calcifications (**b**) are present outside the mass, suggesting the presence of carcinoma.

Comment: In other cases, noninfiltrating papillary carcinoma cannot be identified or cannot be differentiated from benign disease on the mammogram.

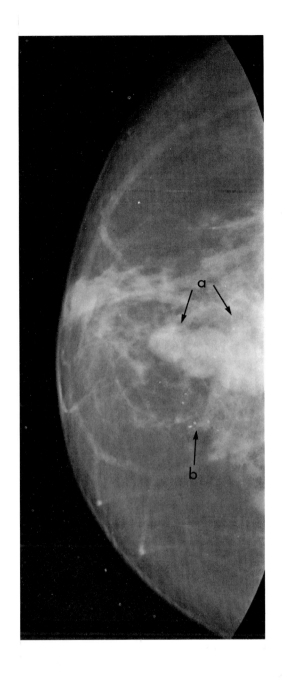

Figure 113 · Noninfiltrating Papillary Carcinoma / 247

Figure 114.—Infiltrating papillary carcinoma.

A 56-year-old woman bled from the right nipple. No definite mass was palpable. Radical mastectomy was performed. Pathologically, the lesion was a multicentric intraductal grade 2 papillary adenocarcinoma with focal infiltration of the periductal stroma. Axillary lymph nodes were free from tumor.

Mammogram, craniocaudal view: A multinodular lesion (**arrows**) involves the central part of the breast beneath the nipple. A few flecks of calcium are present, but these are not a prominent part of the process. Some of the nodules have irregular margins suggesting invasive tumor; however, most appear as nodular dilatations of ducts.

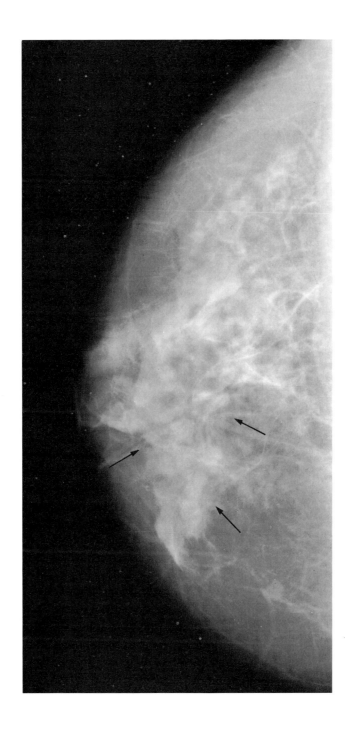

Figure 114 · **Infiltrating Papillary Carcinoma** / **249**

Figure 115.—Infiltrating papillary carcinoma: variations in appearance.

A, mammogram, mediolateral view: Multiple nodules (**arrows**) are seen. Most are well circumscribed, and the largest is lobulated, suggesting fibroadenoma. Retraction of the nipple is present.

Because of the mass in the right breast of this 81-year-old woman, simple mastectomy was performed. Pathologically, the lesion was a multicentric grade 2 papillary carcinoma with some areas of comedocarcinoma. The largest nodule measured 3 cm in its greatest diameter.

B, mammogram, mediolateral view: Two well-circumscribed nodules (**a**) are seen immediately beneath the areola, with an irregular invasive-appearing area (**b**) deeper in the breast. This lesion is difficult to distinguish from fibrocystic disease.

A multinodular mass was palpable beneath the nipple of one breast of this 81-year-old woman. Simple mastectomy was performed. Pathologically, the lesion was a multicentric grade 2 papillary carcinoma with associated areas of comedo- and scirrhous carcinoma.

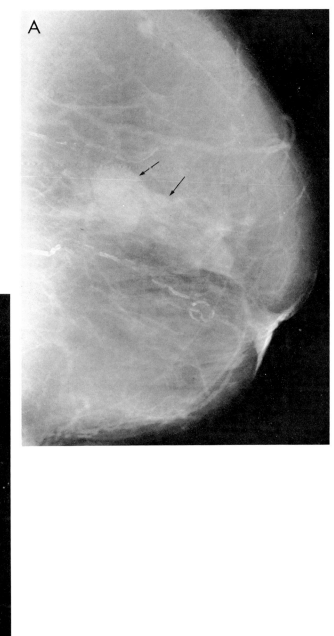

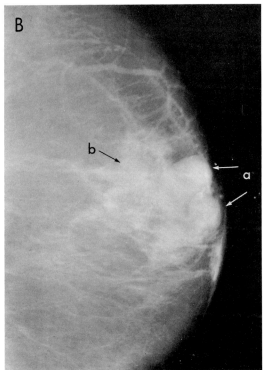

Figure 115 · **Infiltrating Papillary Carcinoma / 251**

Figure 116.—Medullary carcinoma: circumscribed type.

A, mammogram, mediolateral view: A tumor fills the entire breast. It is well circumscribed and homogeneous in density. No evidence of invasion of surrounding tissue is seen, and the overlying skin of the breast is normal.

Clinically, this 83-year-old woman had a large mass filling the entire left breast. The lesion was freely movable and no skin changes suggesting carcinoma were present. Radical mastectomy was performed. Pathologically, the lesion was a circumscribed medullary adenocarcinoma, 8.5 cm in diameter. There was extensive central necrosis with cyst formation. Axillary nodes were not involved.

B, localized section of a mammogram: Showing a tumor that is fairly well circumscribed, but with evidence of invasion along its posterior and superior margins (**arrows**).

The 62-year-old woman had had a slowly enlarging mass in the breast for at least 1 year. The lesion was soft and freely movable. Radical mastectomy was performed. Pathologically, the lesion was a grade 3 medullary adenocarcinoma, 3.5 cm in diameter. Axillary lymph nodes were free from tumor.

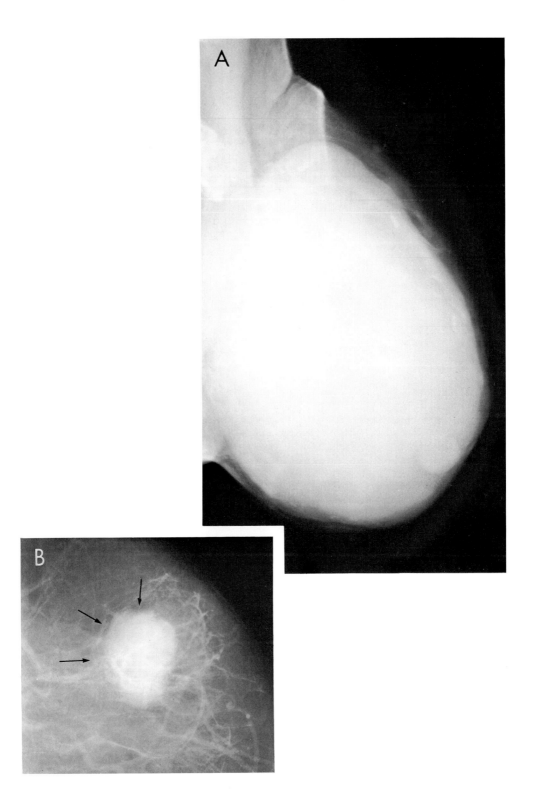

Figure 116 · Medullary Carcinoma: Circumscribed Type / 253

Figure 117.—Medullary carcinoma: diffuse type.

A 64-year-old woman had a palpable mass in the right breast, which was clinically indeterminate. Radical mastectomy was performed. Pathologically, the lesion was a diffuse grade 4 medullary carcinoma measuring 7 × 6 × 4 cm. One axillary lymph node was metastatically involved by tumor.

A, right breast, mediolateral view: The mammogram shows a diffuse increase of density with some disorder of the architectural pattern. (A lead shot indicates the location of the mass.) It is difficult to determine from this film that a mass is present.

B, left breast, mediolateral view: The normal breast, shown for comparison.

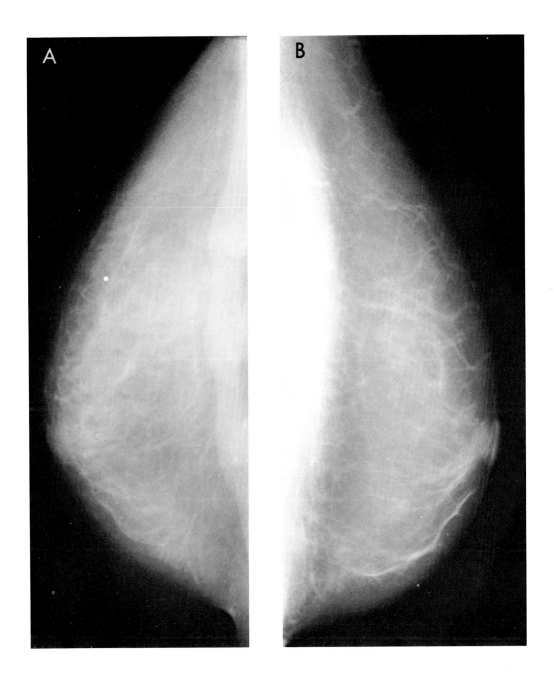

Figure 117 · Medullary Carcinoma: Diffuse Type / 255

Figure 118.—Colloid (mucinous) carcinoma.

A 74-year-old woman had a well-circumscribed nodule in the lower inner quadrant of the left breast. Radical mastectomy was performed. Pathologically, the lesion was an encapsulated grade 2 mucinous adenocarcinoma, 1.5 cm in diameter. Axillary lymph nodes were not involved by metastatic tumor.

A, entire breast, craniocaudal view: A well-circumscribed, slightly lobular tumor is present in the inner aspect of the breast (**arrow**). At first glance, the lesion appears benign, but close scrutiny of the margins reveals evidence of invasive tumor.

B, enlarged segment of the mammogram: This demonstrates the lack of circumscription and the indistinct infiltrative margin of the lesion.

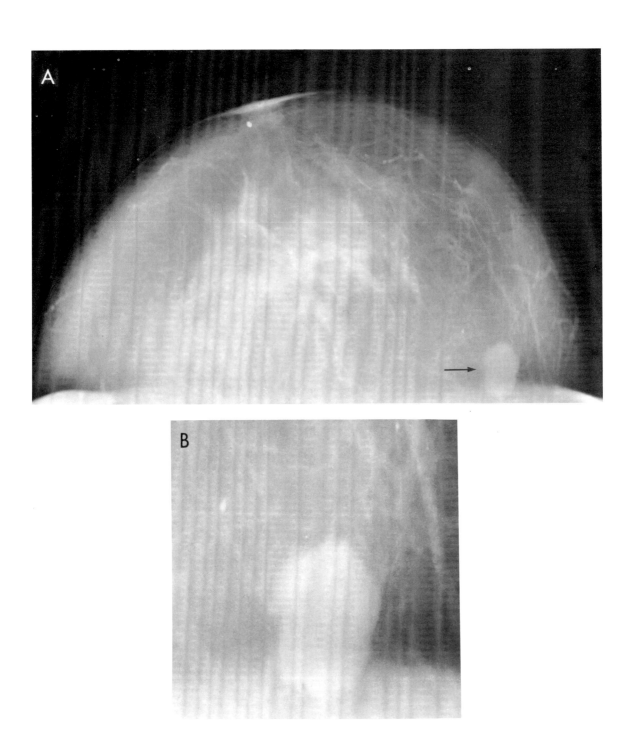

Figure 118 · Colloid Carcinoma / 257

Figure 119.—Colloid (mucinous) carcinoma: circumscribed types.

A, a large opaque tumor with lobular margin and little evidence of invasion at its margins is evident on a mammogram of a 74-year-old woman. Pathologically, the lesion was a grade 2 mucinous adenocarcinoma. There was no axillary lymph node metastasis.

B, a multinodular tumor in the subareolar position is evident in a mammogram of a 68-year-old woman. The margins are sharply circumscribed and the tumor is homogeneous in density. No secondary signs of carcinoma are present. Pathologically, the lesion was a grade 3 mucinous adenocarcinoma. There was no axillary lymph node metastasis.

C, a small well-circumscribed tumor mimics a cyst of fibrocystic disease on a mammogram of a 71-year-old woman. Most of the margin is well defined, but posteriorly (**arrow**), invasive tumor is seen. Nipple retraction and slight thickening of the skin of the nipple are present. Pathologically, the lesion was an encapsulated grade 2 mucinous adenocarcinoma.

Comment: Well-circumscribed mucinous carcinomas of the type illustrated here are difficult to distinguish from benign lesions such as cyst and fibroadenoma.

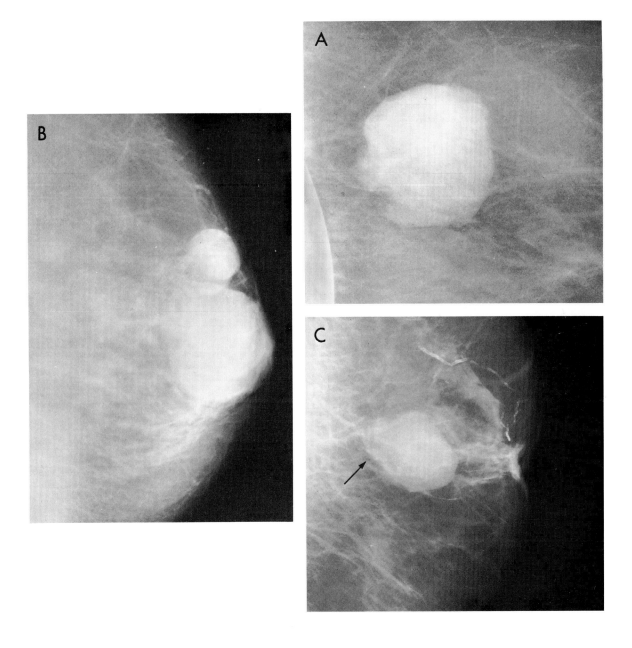

Figure 119 · Colloid Carcinoma: Circumscribed Types / 259

Figure 120.—Colloid (mucinous) carcinoma: diffuse type.

A 48-year-old woman had a fixed mass in the upper outer quadrant of the left breast and palpable left axillary lymphadenopathy. Clinically, the patient had carcinoma. Radical mastectomy was performed. Pathologically, the lesion was a grade 3 mucinous adenocarcinoma measuring 4 cm in its greatest diameter. No metastasis was found in the axillary lymph nodes.

A, mammogram, mediolateral view: There is a large mass with irregular, ill-defined margins in the upper part of the breast (**arrows**). The lesion is partially obscured by dense overlying glandular tissue.

B, enlarged localized view: This shows the tumor in better detail.

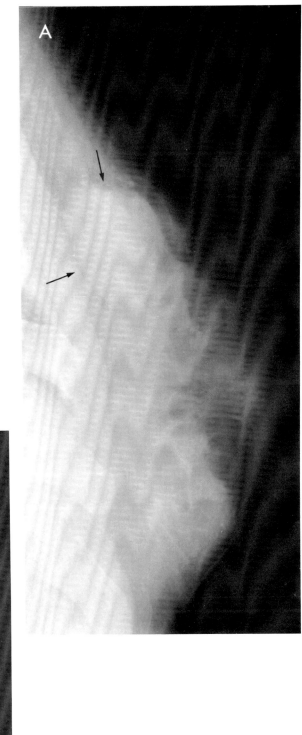

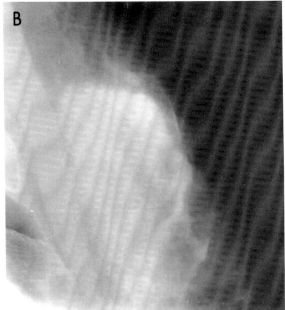

Figure 120 · Colloid Carcinoma: Diffuse Type / 261

Figure 121.—Colloid (mucinous) carcinoma with calcification.

A, mammogram, craniocaudal view made with cassette cut to fit the chest wall: The breast is extremely dense and the tumor is obscured. Coarse irregular calcifications (**arrows**) are present throughout the tumor.

Clinically, a large fixed mass was evident in the upper outer quadrant of the left breast of a 52-year-old woman. Multiple enlarged lymph nodes were palpable in the left axilla. The diagnosis was carcinoma, and a radical mastectomy was performed. Pathologically, the lesion was mucinous adenocarcinoma involving a large region in the upper outer quadrant of the breast. Many coarse calcifications were present in the tumor. Multiple axillary lymph nodes were involved metastatically.

B, a portion of a mammogram: Showing two types of carcinoma distinctly different in appearance. The mucinous tumor (**a**) is circumscribed and contains a few coarse calcifications. The scirrhous tumor (**b**) has typical stellate spicules radiating outward from its margins.

Clinically, two masses were palpable in the right breast of the 77-year-old woman. Diagnosis was carcinoma and a radical mastectomy was performed. Pathologically, there were two separate primary tumors, one a grade 2 mucinous carcinoma and the other a grade 3 scirrhous carcinoma. Multiple axillary lymph nodes were involved by metastatic tumor.

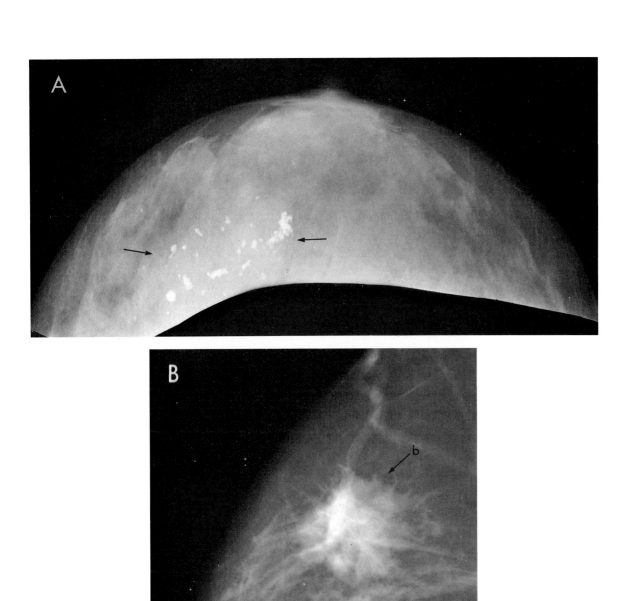

Figure 121 · Colloid Carcinoma: With Calcification / 263

Figure 122.—Noninfiltrating lobular carcinoma (lobular carcinoma in situ).

A, localized enlarged portion of a mammogram: There is a small cluster of punctate calcifications (**arrow**) in an area of lobular carcinoma in situ. No mass was palpable. Biopsy was performed on the basis of the mammographic detection of this calcification.

B, localized enlarged segment of a mammogram: Two small clusters of calcification (**arrows**) represent a region containing foci of both lobular carcinoma in situ and intraductal carcinoma.

Comment: Lobular carcinoma in situ is almost always found in breasts containing large amounts of dense glandular tissue. Calcifications of the type illustrated here are found in approximately half of the cases and, while not pathognomonic of the disease, are strongly suggestive. When calcifications of this type are identified, biopsy is indicated.

Figure 122, courtesy of Snyder, R. E.: Surg., Gynec. & Obst. 122:255-260, 1966.

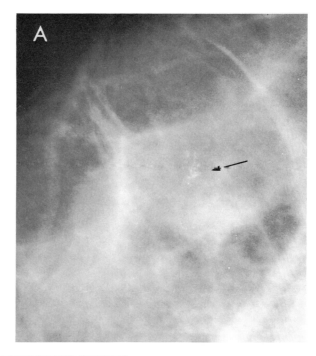

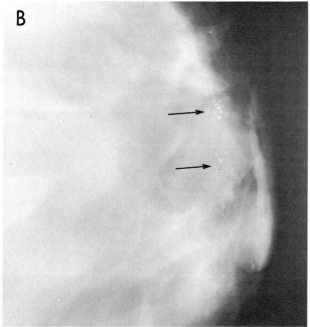

Figure 122 · Noninfiltrating Lobular Carcinoma / 265

Figure 123.—Infiltrating lobular carcinoma.

A 68-year-old woman had a palpable mass in the midportion of the left breast. A radical mastectomy was performed. Pathologically, the lesion was a multicentric infiltrating grade 4 lobular carcinoma forming two separate discrete nodules, the larger one 3 cm in diameter. There were associated foci of in situ grade 4 lobular carcinoma. Axillary and internal mammary lymph nodes were free from tumor.

A, left breast, craniocaudal view: A poorly defined stellate mass (**arrows**) of low radiographic density is present in the midportion of the breast. The spiculation of the margins is typical of carcinoma. Increased vascularity with enlargement of the veins is present. A single rounded, benign-appearing calcification is seen lateral to the tumor.

B, right breast, craniocaudal view, for comparison: There is some residual subareolar fibrosis (**a**) with coarse benign calcification.

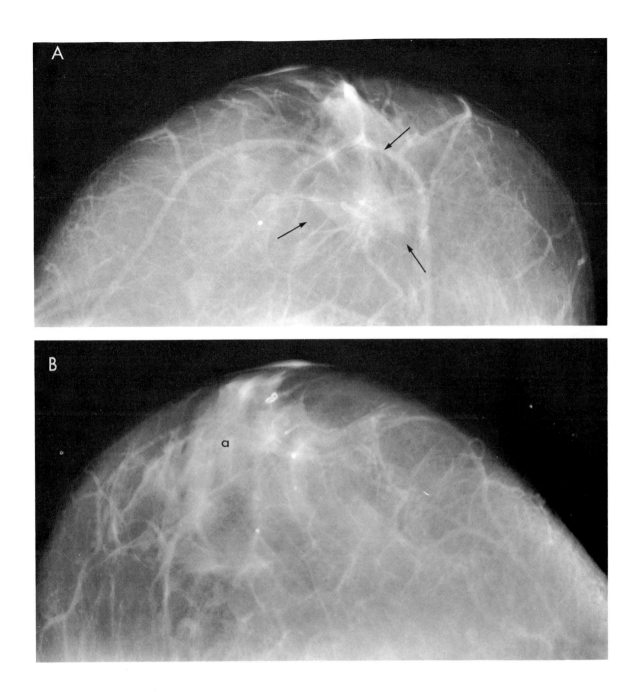

Figure 123 · Infiltrating Lobular Carcinoma / 267

Figure 124.—Infiltrating mixed lobular and comedocarcinoma.

A 44-year-old woman had a palpable mass in the lower portion of the right breast below the nipple. Axillary lymph nodes were palpable bilaterally. A radical mastectomy was performed. Pathologically, the lesion was a multicentric infiltrating grade 3 lobular and comedocarcinoma forming a mass 4 cm in greatest diameter. Axillary lymph nodes contained lymphoma of the giant follicular type.

A, mammogram, mediolateral view: The breast is of the glandular type and is very opaque. A localized area of finely stippled calcification (**arrows**) is present below the nipple in the lower part of the breast. No associated mass is seen.

B, localized view to show calcifications (**arrows**) in better detail: These are numerous, punctate and angular.

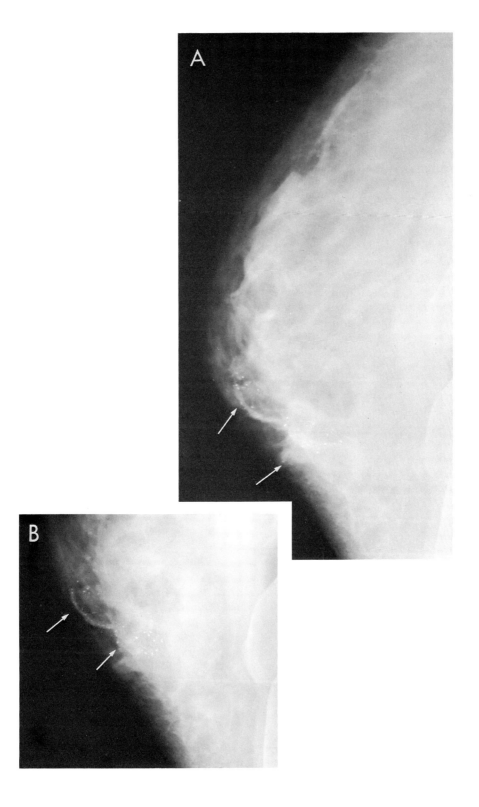

Figure 124 · Infiltrating Lobular and Comedocarcinoma / 269

Figure 125.—Paget's disease.

A 62-year-old woman had a serous discharge from the right nipple and minimal eczematoid changes in the skin of the nipple. No mass was palpable. A radical mastectomy was performed. Pathologically, the lesion was an intraepithelial adenocarcinoma (Paget's disease) with an underlying focus of grade 3 adenocarcinoma, 0.3 cm in diameter, involving the mammary ducts approximately 5 cm from the nipple. Axillary lymph nodes were free from metastatic carcinoma.

A, right breast, craniocaudal view: The skin of the nipple and areola (**arrows**) is thickened, and there is slight flattening of the areolar tissues. The underlying carcinoma in the mammary ducts cannot be identified.

B, left breast, craniocaudal view: Normal breast, shown for comparison.

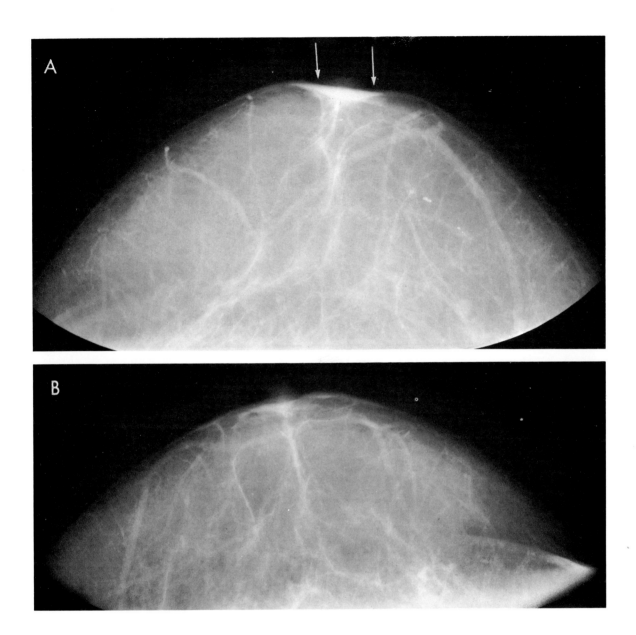

Figure 125 · Paget's Disease / 271

Figure 126.—Paget's disease: variations in radiographic appearance.

A, mammogram, craniocaudal view: There is an ill-defined invasive mass (**a**) in the lateral aspect of the breast, with thickening of the skin of the nipple and areola (**b**).

The 68-year-old patient had eczematoid changes of the nipple and a palpable mass in the lateral aspect of the left breast. A radical mastectomy was performed. Pathologically, the lesion was a grade 4 comedocarcinoma, 2.5 cm in diameter, with an intraepithelial extension into the nipple (Paget's disease). Axillary lymph nodes were normal.

B, a portion of a mammogram: A typical invasive carcinoma (**a**) is present in the subareolar position. The lesion is heavily calcified. No changes in the nipple (**b**) are seen.

This 58-year-old woman had a mass near the areola of one breast. A radical mastectomy was performed. Pathologically, there was Paget's disease of the nipple with underlying grade 4 scirrhous adenocarcinoma. In situ carcinoma extended along a single duct from the primary tumor to the nipple.

C, mammogram, mediolateral view: The nipple (**a**) is retracted and thickened. There are extensive tumor calcification (**b**) and fibrosis throughout the central portion of the breast.

This 54-year-old woman had ulceration of the nipple and a mass in the breast. A radical mastectomy was performed. Pathologically, there was Paget's disease of the nipple with diffuse multicentric grade 4 comedocarcinoma extensively involving the breast. Aside from the invasion of the nipple, the carcinoma did not seem to extend beyond the thickened ducts.

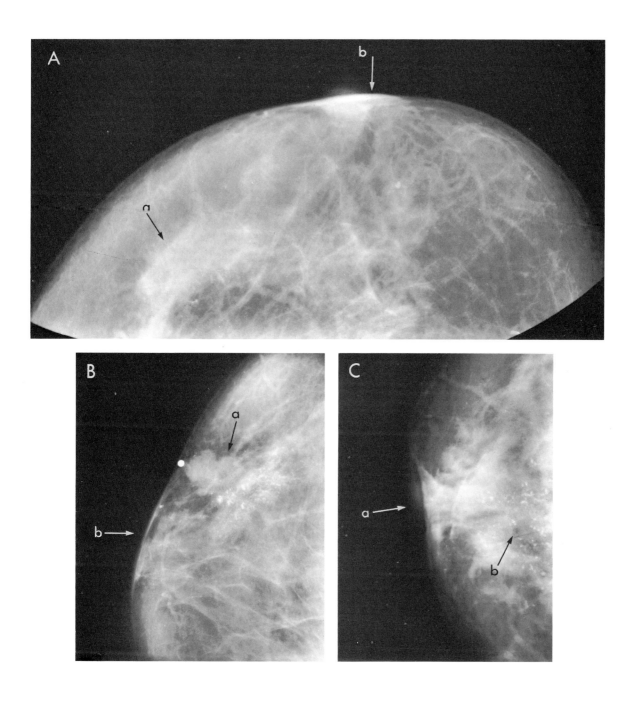

Figure 126 · **Paget's Disease: Variations in Appearance / 273**

Figure 127.—Intracystic carcinoma.

A 72-year-old woman had a well-circumscribed mass beneath the right nipple. The lesion was clinically benign. Simple mastectomy was performed. Pathologically, the lesion was an infiltrating grade 1 papillary cystadeno-carcinoma with a cyst 2.5 cm in diameter and an intramural nodule of tumor 1 cm in diameter. In the lateral aspect of the breast were a number of active benign intraductal papillomas measuring 1–0.3 cm in diameter.

Mammogram, craniocaudal view: This shows a well-circumscribed but somewhat irregular mass (**a**) immediately beneath the areola. The irregularity of the deep surface of the mass suggests invasion by tumor in this area. Multiple discrete nodular densities (**b**) in the lateral part of the breast represent the benign papillomas found in the specimen. The nature of these lesions cannot be deduced from their radiographic appearance.

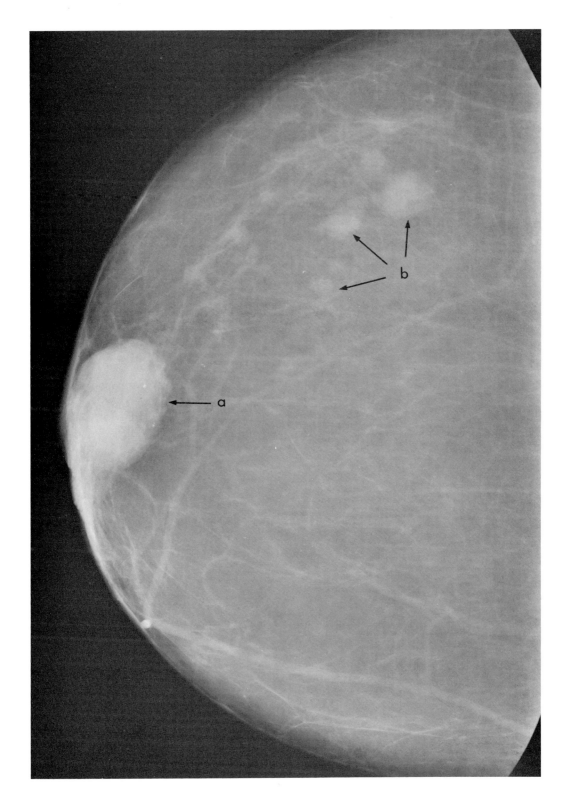

Figure 127 · Intracystic Carcinoma / 275

Figure 128.—Intracystic carcinoma.

A, mammogram, craniocaudal view: There is a large smooth-walled mass with a small lobular projection on its posterolateral wall (**arrow**). The sharp circumscription of the wall and the absence of signs of invasive tumor give this lesion a benign appearance.

A 78-year-old woman had a large cystic mass in the right breast. The lesion had increased rapidly in size in the weeks prior to examination. Simple mastectomy was performed. Pathologically, there was a grade 2 papillary adenocarcinoma in the wall of a large cyst filled with hemorrhagic fluid. The tumor was invasive and measured 2 cm in diameter.

B, mammogram, mediolateral view: A lesion (**arrows**) is partially obscured by overlying breast tissue, but where seen, it appears to be well circumscribed. Multiple punctate calcifications are present, suggesting the malignant nature of the disease.

A 65-year-old woman had a small cystic mass in the left breast. A radical mastectomy was performed. Pathologically, there was an intracystic grade 2 papillary adenocarcinoma 1 cm in diameter in the wall of a cyst measuring 2 cm in diameter. Axillary lymph nodes were normal.

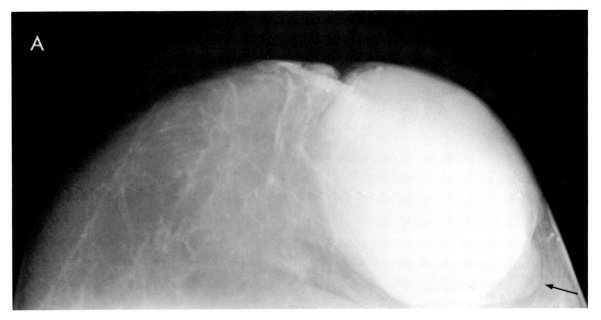

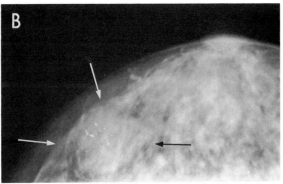

Figure 128 · Intracystic Carcinoma / 277

Figure 129.—Apocrine "sweat gland" carcinoma.

A 55-year-old woman had a hard mass in the lateral aspect of the right breast. A radical mastectomy was performed. Pathologically, the lesion was a grade 3 infiltrating apocrine sweat gland carcinoma. Axillary lymph nodes were free from tumor.

Mammogram, mediolateral view: The breast is seen to contain a large amount of dense glandular tissue which partially obscures the carcinoma. The lesion (**arrows**), which lies in the lateral aspect of the breast, disrupts the architectural pattern and is irregular in outline. On the original radiograph, fine spicules of invasive tumor could be identified. The veins in the region of the lesion are enlarged, indicating an increase of blood flow. No features differentiate this lesion from other types of carcinoma.

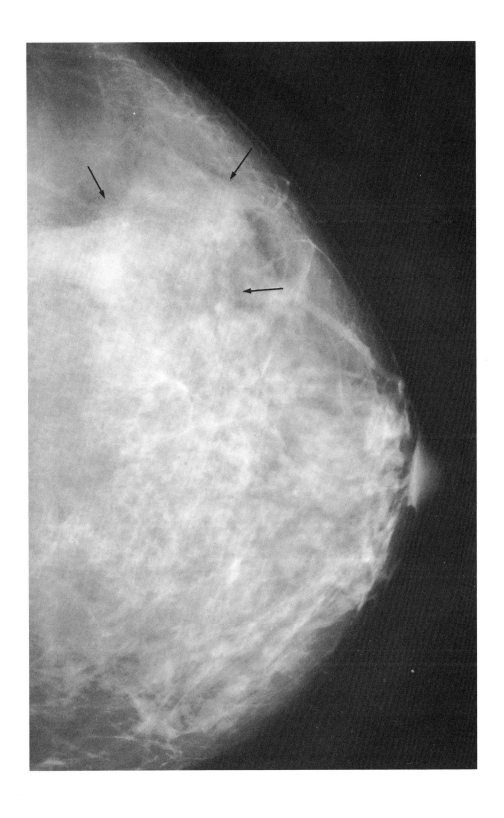

Figure 129 · Apocrine "Sweat Gland" Carcinoma / 279

Figure 130.—Adenoid cystic carcinoma (cylindroma).

On physical examination of a 70-year-old woman, an ill-defined nodular lesion was found in the upper outer quadrant of the right breast. A radical mastectomy was performed. Pathologically, the lesion was a grade 2 adenocarcinoma of the adenoid cystic (cylindroma) type. The lesion measured roughly 2.5 cm in diameter. Axillary lymph nodes were normal.

A, mammogram, mediolateral view: An irregular lesion (**arrow**) in the upper part of the breast suggests thickened ducts and residual glandular structures. A few flecks of calcium are present within the lesion. No similar density was present in the opposite breast.

B, enlarged segment of the mammogram to show detailed appearance of the lesion: The margins are indistinct and the tumor is not homogeneous in density. Several small calcifications (**arrow**) are present, some of which appear rounded.

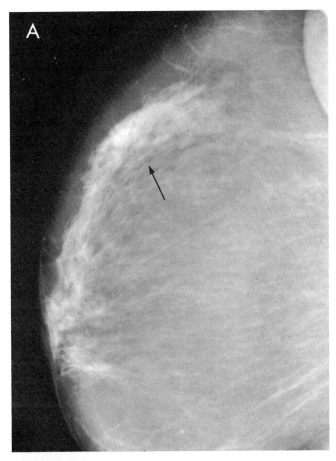

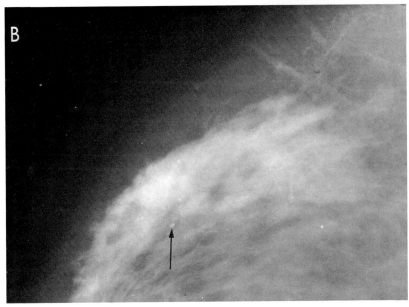

Figure 130 · Adenoid Cystic Carcinoma (Cylindroma) / 281

Figure 131.—Multicentric carcinoma.

A 58-year-old woman had multiple small palpable nodules in one breast. A radical mastectomy was performed. Pathologically, the nodules represented multicentric grade 3 scirrhous adenocarcinoma. Multiple separate nodules, up to 1.5 cm in diameter, were scattered throughout the breast. Axillary lymph nodes were not involved.

Mammogram, craniocaudal view: At least eight separate deposits of tumor (**a**) are seen. Each of these has the typical stellate appearance of scirrhous carcinoma. Localized skin thickening (**b**) is present over the largest lesion, which lies in a subcutaneous position on the lateral aspect of the breast.

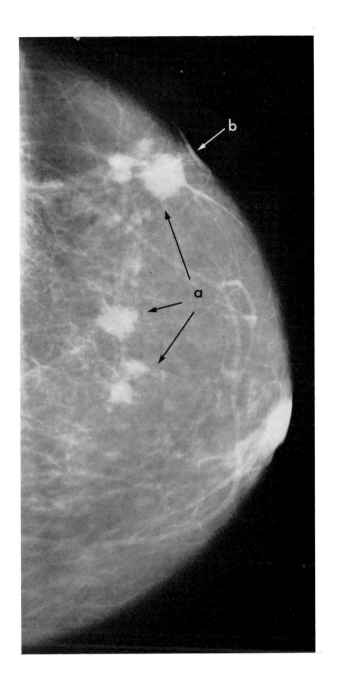

Figure 131 · Multicentric Carcinoma / 283

Figure 132.—Multicentric carcinoma.

A 77-year-old woman had two distinct palpable masses in the left breast. A radical mastectomy was performed. Pathologically, two carcinomas, one a grade 2 mucinous adenocarcinoma 1.5 cm in diameter and the other a grade 1 infiltrating papillary carcinoma 1.5 cm in diameter, were separated by approximately 5 cm of normal breast tissue. Axillary lymph nodes were normal.

Mammogram, craniocaudal view: Two circumscribed lesions (**arrows**) are present in the medial aspect of the breast. Both are irregular in outline with indistinct margins due to invasion of surrounding tissues. On the original film, fine calcifications could be seen in both lesions.

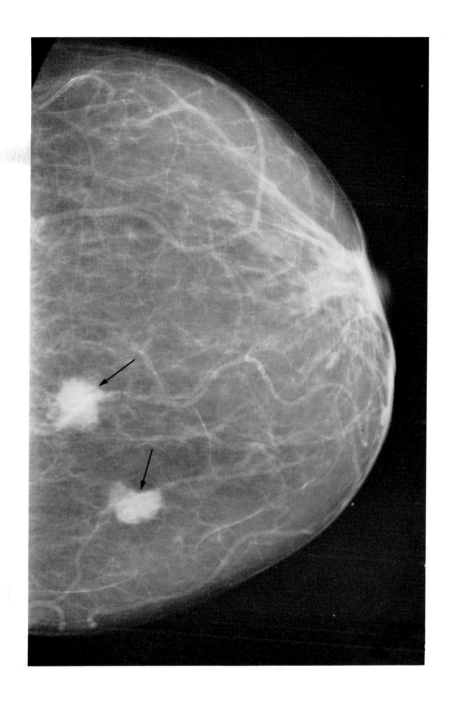

Figure 132 · Multicentric Carcinoma / 285

Figure 133.—Simultaneous bilateral carcinoma.

A palpable mass in the left breast of a woman, 63, was thought to be a carcinoma. No mass was palpable in the right breast. Bilateral radical mastectomy was performed. Pathologically, there were bilateral primary carcinomas. The left breast contained a 3-cm, grade 4 scirrhous adenocarcinoma; there was metastasis to a single lymph node. The right breast con-

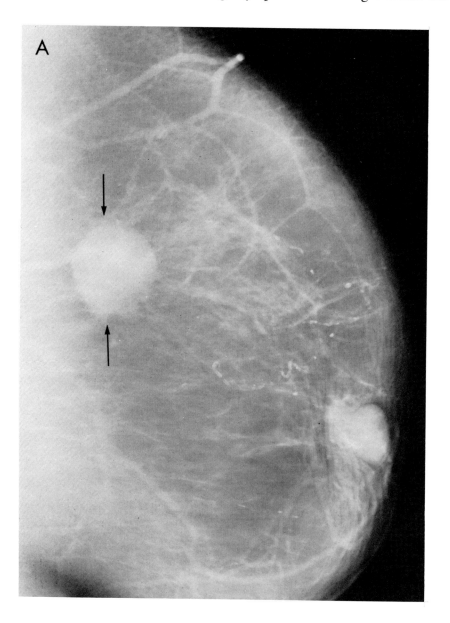

tained a 1.5-cm, grade 3 intraductal (comedo) infiltrative adenocarcinoma; axillary lymph nodes were normal.

A, left breast, mediolateral view: A large circumscribed tumor (**arrows**) in the upper outer quadrant has stellate margins typical of carcinoma.

B, right breast, mediolateral view: A small irregular, poorly defined infiltrating tumor (**arrows**) above the nipple contains fine flecks of calcium.

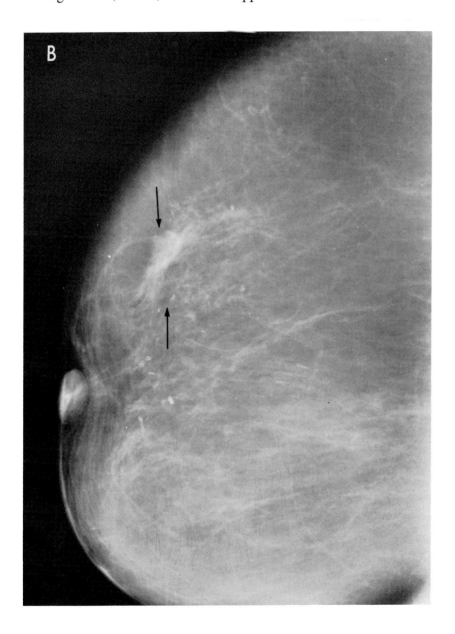

Figure 133 · **Simultaneous Bilateral Carcinoma** / **287**

Figure 134.—Simultaneous bilateral carcinoma.

A 64-year-old woman had a large hard mass typical of carcinoma in the right breast. No lesion was palpable in the left breast. Bilateral radical mastectomy was performed. Pathologically, the right breast contained a diffuse infiltrating grade 4 scirrhous adenocarcinoma involving the central portion of the breast; multiple axillary lymph nodes were involved metastatically. The left breast contained a grade 3 scirrhous adenocarcinoma 1.5 cm in diameter, which probably was a second primary; axillary lymph nodes were normal.

A, right breast, craniocaudal view: A large infiltrating tumor fills the central part of the breast. There are retraction of the nipple (**arrow**), thickening of the skin over the medial half of the breast and disruption of the architectural pattern of the parenchyma.

B, left breast, craniocaudal view: A small circumscribed, poorly marginated tumor (**arrow**), typical of carcinoma, is present in the lateral aspect of the breast.

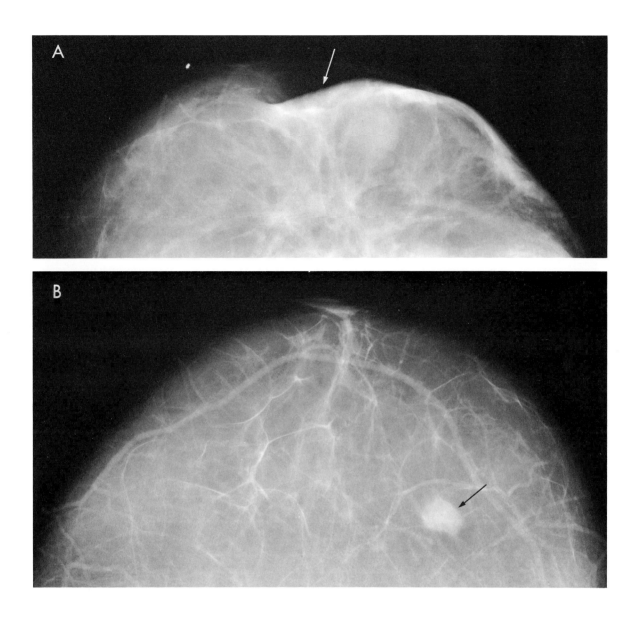

Figure 134 · Simultaneous Bilateral Carcinoma / 289

Figure 135.—Metastatic carcinoma of remaining breast after mastectomy: diffuse type.

A 36-year-old woman had had left mastectomy for carcinoma. The right breast had been clinically and radiographically normal at the time of the initial operation (**A**). Diffuse metastasis developed in the lungs and in the remaining breast within 1 year (**B**). Biopsy of the right breast revealed diffuse metastatic adenocarcinoma.

A, uninvolved right breast at time of initial operation, mediolateral view: There is considerable dense glandular tissue which is normal in appearance. No evidence of carcinoma is seen.

B, right breast 1 year after left mastectomy for carcinoma, mediolateral view: Diffuse thickening and deformity of the skin (**arrows**) as well as disruption of the architectural pattern of the breast parenchyma have developed. The appearance is typical of diffuse metastatic carcinoma.

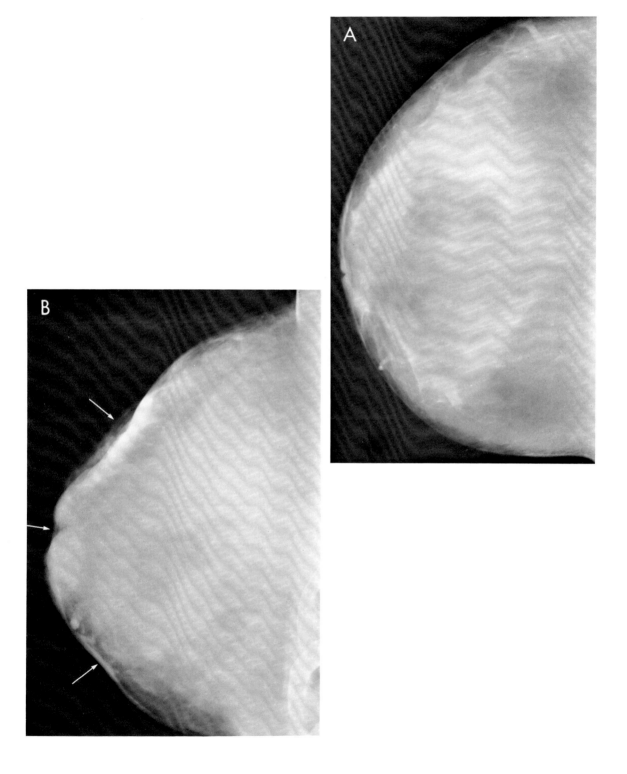

Figure 135 · Carcinoma of Remaining Breast: Metastatic / 291

Figure 136.—Metastatic carcinoma of remaining breast after mastectomy: localized type.

A 72-year-old woman had mastectomy of the right breast for carcinoma. Follow-up examination 18 months after operation revealed a mass in the left breast which had not been present on mammograms made at the time of right mastectomy. The lesion was clinically palpable and was considered to be a metastasis. Nodular metastasis was present in the lungs. Biopsy was not performed.

Mammogram of the remaining left breast, craniocaudal view: There is a circumscribed lesion (**arrow**), 2.5 cm in diameter, with invasive margins characteristic of carcinoma.

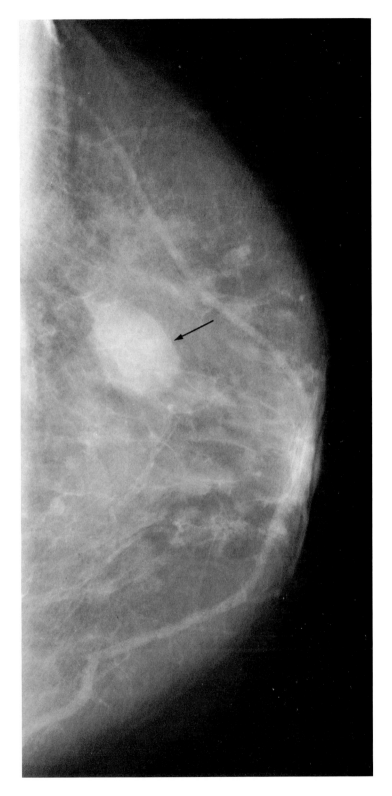

Figure 136 · Carcinoma of Remaining Breast: Metastatic / 293

Figure 137.—Carcinoma of remaining breast after mastectomy: new primary.

A 70-year-old woman had had left radical mastectomy for carcinoma of the breast 9 years previously. Routine physical examination revealed no new findings. No mass was palpable in the remaining breast, but mammography revealed a small tumor. Right radical mastectomy was performed. Pathologically, the lesion was a primary grade 3 scirrhous adenocarcinoma 0.8 cm in diameter. Axillary lymph nodes were normal.

Mammogram, craniocaudal view: A tiny stellate carcinoma is seen in the lateral aspect of the breast (**a**). Several small collections of benign-appearing calcifications are scattered in the central part of the breast (**b**).

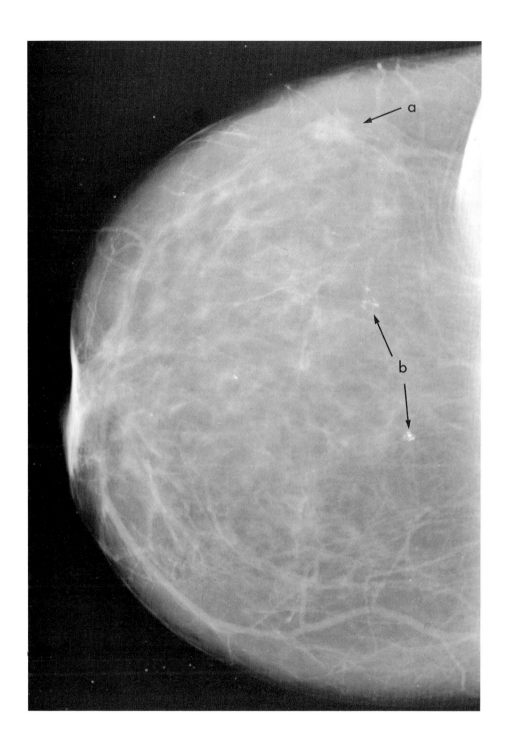

Figure 137 · Carcinoma of Remaining Breast: New Primary / 295

Figure 138.—Carcinoma of remaining breast after mastectomy: new primary.

A 50-year-old woman had had left mastectomy for carcinoma 4 years previously. The initial lesion was a mixed comedo- and scirrhous carcinoma, and systemic metastasis had developed shortly after the operation. The metastatic tumor responded unusually well to palliative therapy. A follow-up mammogram 4 years after the initial operation (**A**) showed a small lesion, not previously present, in the right breast. Re-examination 8 months later demonstrated growth of the lesion. Simple mastectomy with removal of axillary nodes (palliative) was performed. Pathologically, the lesion was a primary grade 3 circumscribed medullary adenocarcinoma. Axillary lymph nodes were free from tumor.

A, mammogram 4 years after initial operation, mediolateral view: A tiny ill-defined density (**arrows**) suggestive of infiltrating carcinoma is seen deep in the central part of the breast.

B, mammogram 8 months later, mediolateral view: The lesion (**arrows**) has more than doubled in size in the interval and is a typical invasive carcinoma.

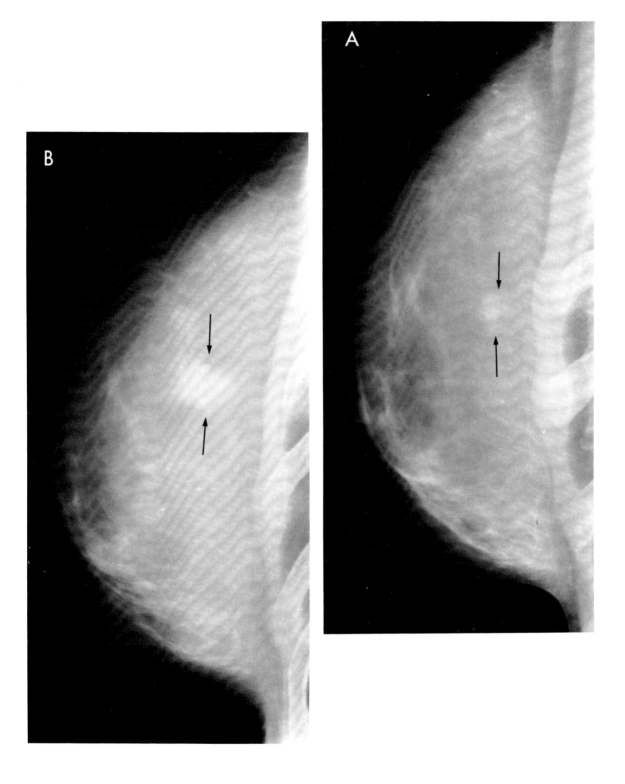

Figure 138 · Carcinoma of Remaining Breast: New Primary / 297

Figure 139.—Carcinoma in pregnancy.

A 50-year-old woman, approximately 4 months pregnant, had a rapidly enlarging mass in the left breast. Clinically, she had carcinoma. Left radical mastectomy, total abdominal hysterectomy and bilateral salpingo-oophorectomy were performed. Pathologically, the mass in the breast was a grade 3 scirrhous adenocarcinoma, 3 cm in diameter. Multiple axillary lymph nodes were involved by metastatic tumor.

Mammogram, mediolateral view: An irregular infiltrative tumor (**a**) with a coarse spiculated margin is present in the upper outer quadrant. Nipple retraction (**b**) is present. The radiographic density of the parenchyma of the breast is considerably less than that usually seen in younger patients during pregnancy.

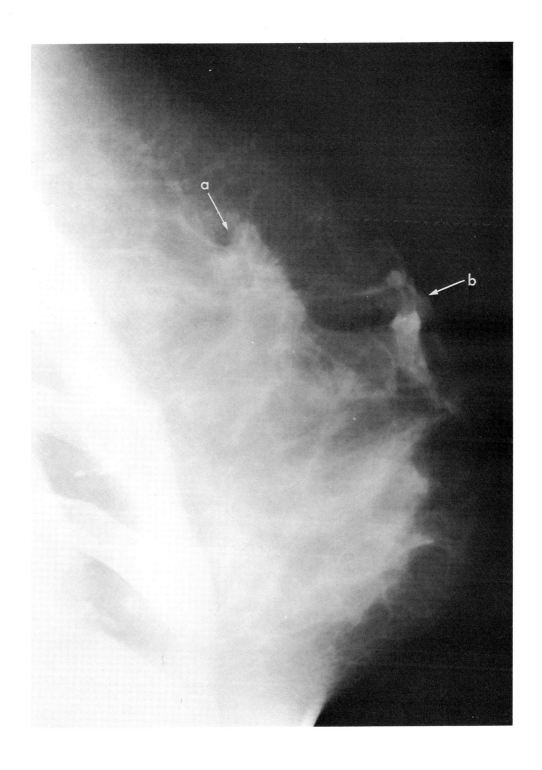

Figure 139 · Carcinoma in Pregnancy / 299

Figure 140.—Carcinoma in pregnancy.

A 30-year-old woman was in the first trimester of pregnancy. A clinically indeterminate palpable mass was found in the upper outer quadrant of the left breast during her initial antepartum examination. A radical mastectomy was performed. Pathologically, the lesion was a grade 4 scirrhous adenocarcinoma, 5.5 cm in diameter. No axillary lymph node metastasis was found.

Mammogram of the left breast, craniocaudal view: A circumscribed mass (**arrows**) is largely obscured by overlying dense breast parenchyma. It is not possible to differentiate accurately between carcinoma and benign tumor in this case.

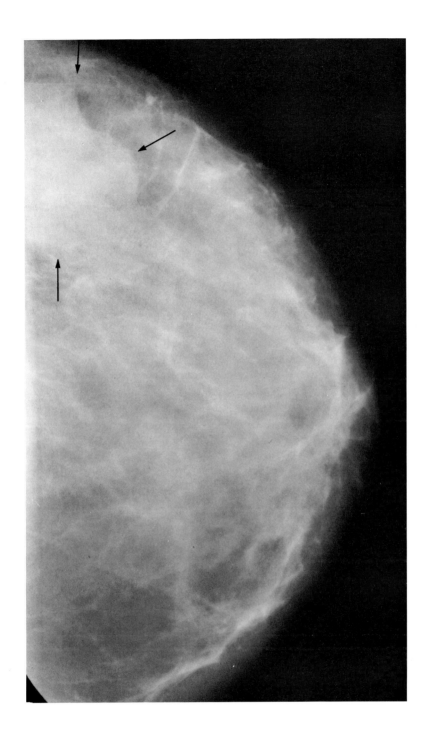

Figure 140 · Carcinoma in Pregnancy / 301

Figure 141.—Carcinoma in pregnancy.

A 36-year-old pregnant woman had clinical signs suggesting either breast abscess or inflammatory carcinoma in the right breast. Radical mastectomy was performed. Pathologically, in addition to the usual changes of the gravid breast, there was an adenocarcinoma in the upper outer quadrant, with intramammary extension of the neoplasm into the subepidermal lymphatics. Of 29 axillary lymph nodes, 28 contained metastatic carcinoma.

A, left breast, craniocaudal view: The normal gravid breast has a diffuse opacity produced by growth of glandular structures.

B, right breast, craniocaudal view: This breast is more opaque than the left, especially in the lateral aspect (**a**). A definite mass suggesting carcinoma is not clearly evident. Diffuse thickening of the skin (**b**) is present, and the architectural pattern of the breast is disrupted. It is not possible to distinguish clearly between breast abscess and diffuse carcinoma.

Figure 141, courtesy of Dr. Donald R. Mueller, Grand Rapids, Minn.

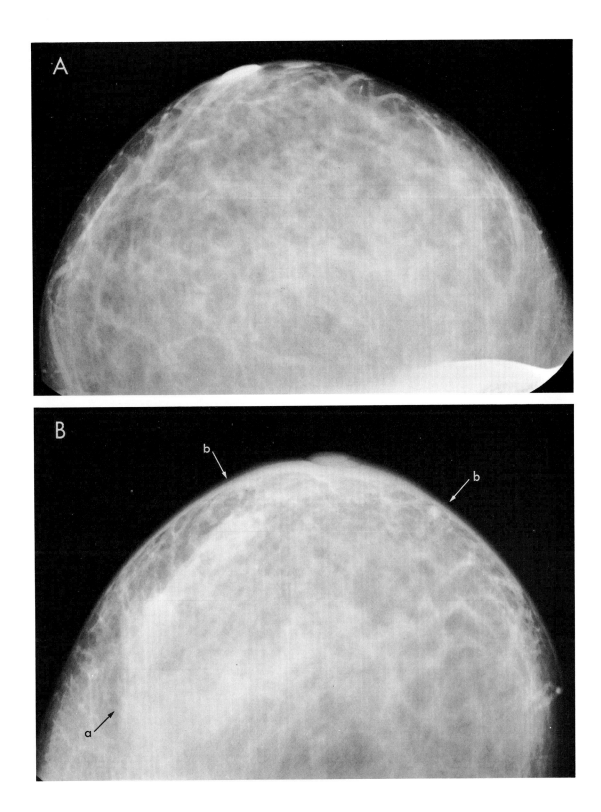

Figure 141 · Carcinoma in Pregnancy / 303

Figure 142.—Carcinoma of the male breast.

A 48-year-old man had a slowly enlarging mass beneath the areola of the left breast. The lesion had been present for at least 6 months. Simple mastectomy and axillary lymph node dissection were performed. Pathologically, the lesion was a grade 4 adenocarcinoma 1.6 cm in diameter. No metastasis was found in the axillary lymph nodes.

Enlarged segment of a mammogram: The circumscribed mass (**a**) has indistinct margins typical of carcinoma. There are associated nipple retraction (**b**) and enlargement of the veins of the breast (**c**).

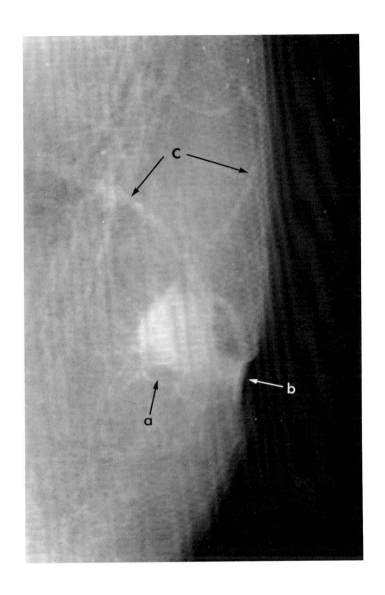

Figure 142 · Carcinoma in Male Breast / 305

Figure 143.—Carcinoma of the male breast with gynecomastia.

A 64-year-old man had carcinoma of the prostate metastatic to bone. Orchiectomy had been performed, and he had received stilbestrol therapy for control of metastasis for 2 years. There had been progressive enlargement of both breasts. A discrete mass in the upper part of the right breast was found on physical examination. A modified radical mastectomy was performed. Pathologically, the lesion was a mixed grade 3 intraductal and scirrhous adenocarcinoma, 2.5 cm in diameter; the breast showed diffuse proliferation and hyperplasia of glandular elements (gynecomastia). Axillary lymph nodes were free from tumor.

A, right breast, mediolateral view: Gynecomastia with marked enlargement of the breast is evident. The parenchyma is very dense. An irregular mass (**arrow**) is present in the upper part of the breast. The stellate sunburst appearance of the lesion is typical of carcinoma.

B, left breast, mediolateral view: The parenchyma is very dense and the breast markedly enlarged. The appearance suggests diffuse fibrocystic disease of the fibrous type.

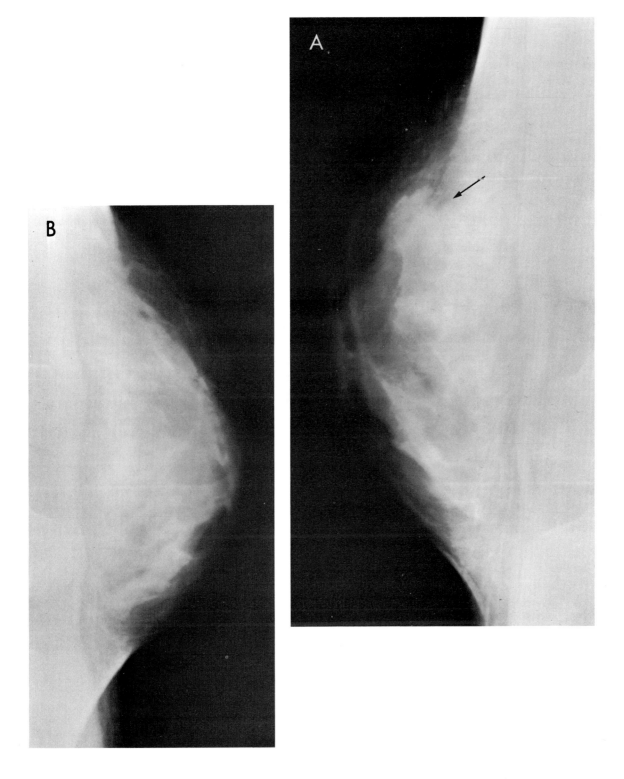

Figure 143 · Carcinoma in Male Breast / 307

Figure 144.—Carcinoma of the male breast simulating gynecomastia.

A 70-year-old man had carcinoma of the prostate. He had had orchiectomy, and there had been slow progressive enlargement of both breasts. A freely movable, firm, clinically benign mass was palpable under the left nipple. Simple mastectomy was performed. Pathologically, the lesion was an encapsulated adenocarcinoma. The pathologist was unable to say whether this was a primary carcinoma of the breast or a metastatic tumor from the prostate.

Mammogram, mediolateral view (enlarged): An irregular nodular lesion (**a**) is situated beneath the nipple (**b**). The appearance of the breast mimics that of gynecomastia, and no definite evidence suggesting carcinoma is seen. The opposite breast, however, was of the fatty type with no radiographic evidence of gynecomastia.

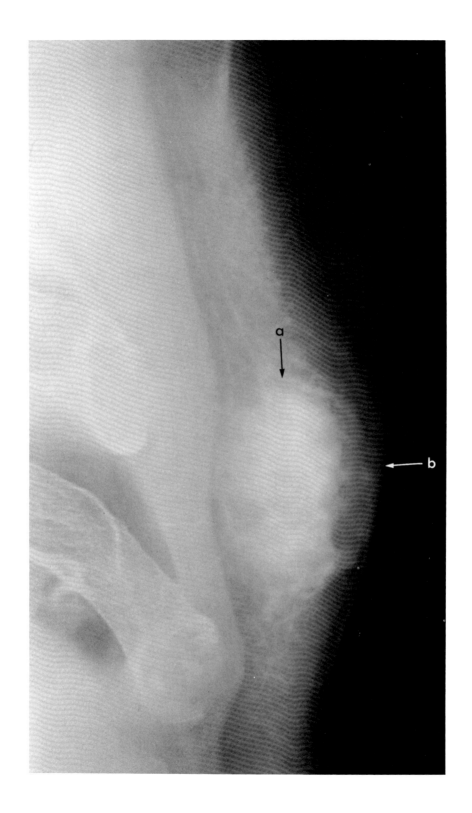

Figure 144 · Carcinoma in Male Breast / 309

Figure 145.—Malignant lymphoma of the breast: circumscribed form.

A 42-year-old woman had lymphosarcoma involving the cervical and mediastinal lymph nodes. A small mass was found in the upper outer quadrant of the left breast. Biopsy demonstrated localized lymphosarcoma.

Mammogram, mediolateral view: A discrete mass with indistinct margins (**arrow**) is seen in the upper outer quadrant of the left breast. No enlarged axillary nodes were visible on the axillary view. The appearance of the lesion suggests well-circumscribed carcinoma.

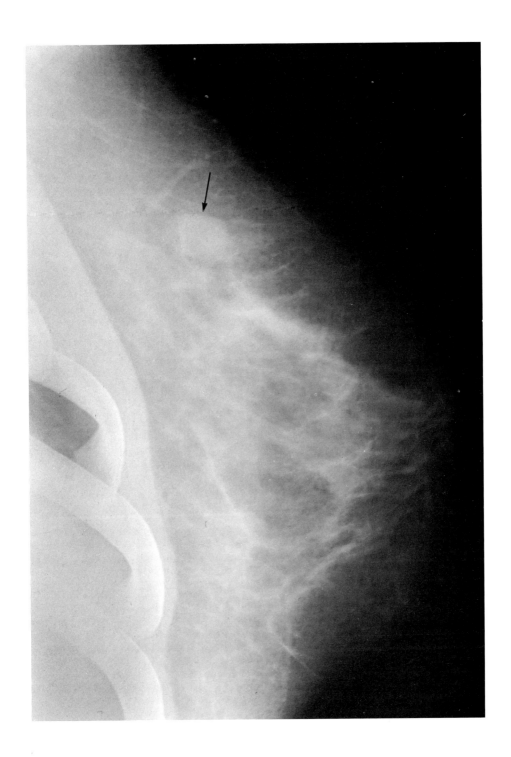

Figure 145 · Malignant Lymphoma: Circumscribed / 311

Figure 146.—Malignant lymphoma, Hodgkin's type, involving the entire breast.

A 44-year-old woman had Hodgkin's disease of the cervical lymph nodes. Recent enlargement of the breast and thickening of the skin had occurred. Biopsy revealed Hodgkin's disease involving the breast.

Mammogram, mediolateral view: There is pronounced disruption of the architectural pattern of the breast with skin thickening (**arrows**) suggestive of diffuse carcinoma. No axillary lymphadenopathy was visible on the axillary view.

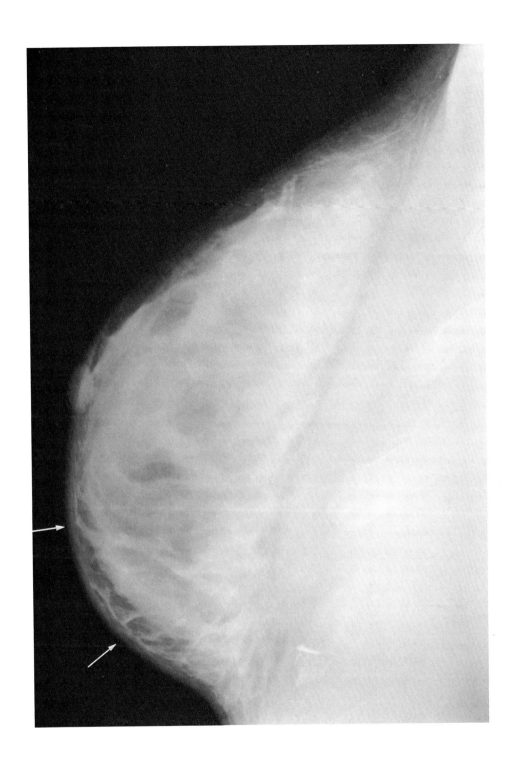

Figure 146 · Malignant Lymphoma: Hodgkin's Type / 313

Figure 147.—Malignant lymphoma of axillary lymph nodes.

A 35-year-old woman had a large fixed mass low in the left axilla. Excisional biopsy of the axillary mass was performed. Pathologically, malignant lymphoma of the lymphocytic type involved a large mass of axillary lymph nodes.

Mammogram, mediolateral view: There is a large well-circumscribed mass (**arrows**) in the tail of the left breast or low in the axilla. The lesion was better demonstrated on this view than on the axillary view. The rest of the breast contained normal-appearing glandular tissue.

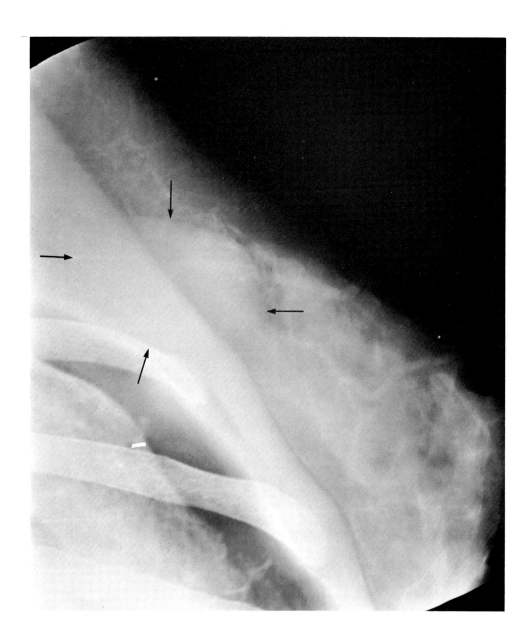

Figure 147 · Malignant Lymphoma / 315

Figure 148.—Malignant lymphoma: lymphatic obstruction with thickening of skin.

A 27-year-old woman had Hodgkin's disease of the axillary and cervical lymph nodes. After irradiation of the involved regions, the breast enlarged and the skin became massively thickened. Biopsy showed lymphedema but no tumor. The edema was apparently secondary to lymphatic obstruction in the axillary and cervical regions.

Mammogram, mediolateral view: The extremely dense breast has an abnormal trabecular pattern and marked thickening of the skin.

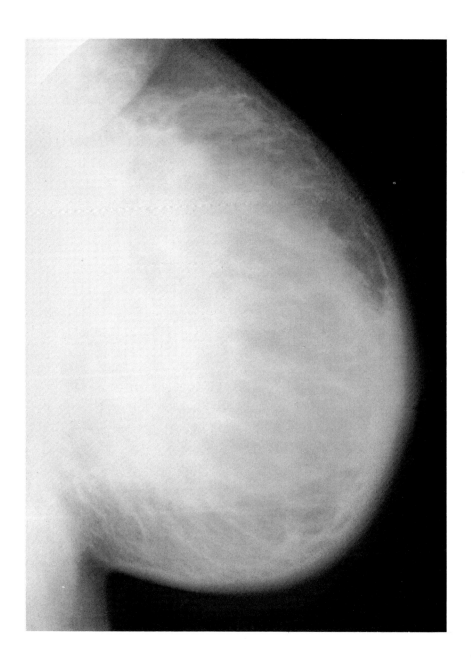

Figure 148 · Malignant Lymphoma / 317

Figure 149.—Malignant melanoma of the nipple.

A 73-year-old woman had an irregular melanotic mass that replaced the nipple of the right breast. Simple mastectomy was performed. Pathologically, the lesion consisted of a malignant melanoma arising in and completely replacing the right nipple. The melanoma extended into the skin adjacent to the nipple for 5 mm.

Mammogram, mediolateral view: The tumor of the nipple (**a**) is nodular and appears almost pedunculated. The skin of the areola (**b**), surrounding the base of the tumor, is thickened by invading tumor.

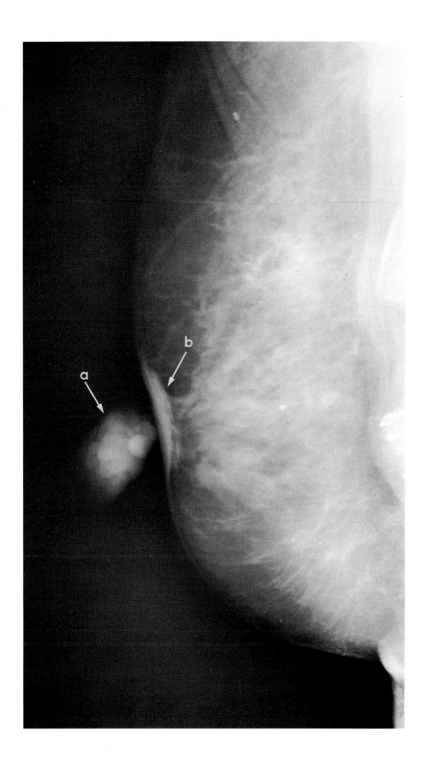

Figure 149 · Malignant Melanoma of Nipple / 319

Figure 150.—Malignant melanoma metastatic to the breast.

A 37-year-old woman had a history of removal of a melanoma from the right leg. Recently multiple nodules had developed at various sites in the body, including both breasts and the abdominal wall. Biopsy revealed metastatic melanoma at all sites.

Mammogram of right breast, craniocaudal view: The two well-circumscribed lesions (**arrows**) have a lobulated appearance suggestive of fibroadenoma. No signs indicate the malignant character of the lesions.

Several smaller nodules of similar character were present in the left breast (not illustrated).

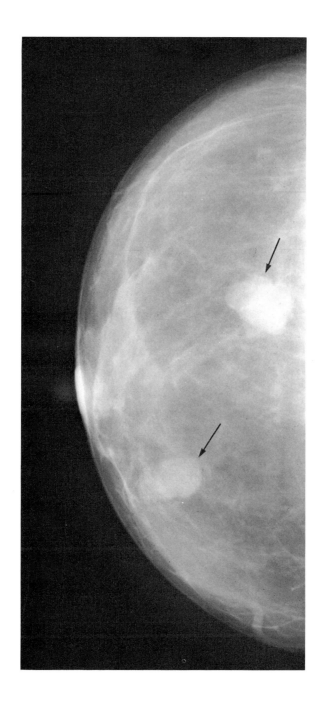

Figure 150 · Malignant Melanoma Metastatic to Breast / 321

Figure 151.—Angiosarcoma.

A 33-year-old woman noticed gradual enlargement of the left breast during a period of several months. A large mass was palpable. Left mastectomy was performed. Pathologically, the lesion was an angiosarcoma 10 cm in its greatest diameter. The tumor was moderately well circumscribed and did not invade overlying skin or the posterior fascia.

A, normal right breast, craniocaudal view: The breast parenchyma is homogeneously dense throughout, suggesting diffuse fibrocystic disease, but the density is not so great nor so homogeneous as that of the left breast.

B, left breast, craniocaudal view: A large homogeneous mass (**arrows**) fills almost the entire breast. Its margins cannot be identified with certainty because of overlying dense glandular tissue. No signs suggesting malignant disease are evident.

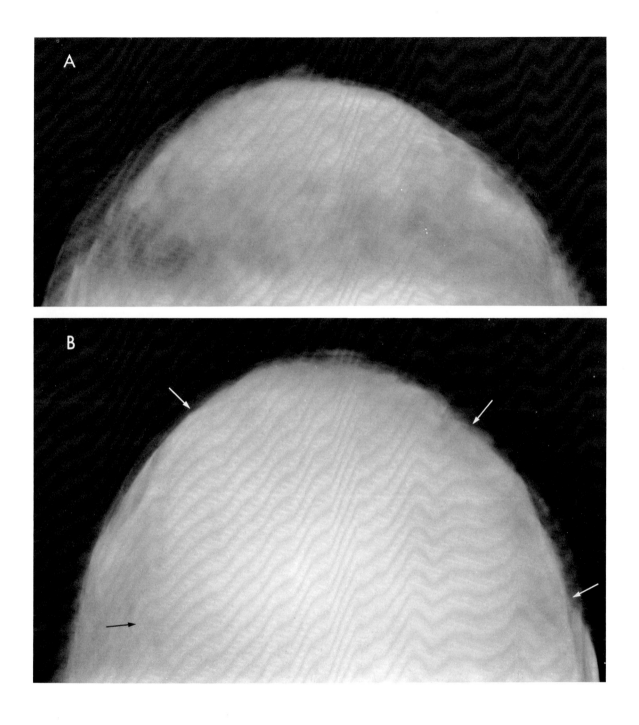

Figure 151 · Angiosarcoma / 323

Figure 152.—Rhabdomyosarcoma.

A 71-year-old woman discovered a mass in the upper outer quadrant of the left breast on self-examination. Clinically, the mass was hard and partially fixed. A radical mastectomy was performed. Pathologically, the lesion was a rhabdomyosarcoma, 3 cm in diameter. Axillary lymph nodes were free from tumor.

Mammogram, mediolateral view: A well-circumscribed lesion (**a**) is situated in the upper outer quadrant of the breast. The margins are somewhat indistinct, suggesting invasive tumor. Several small nodules (**b**) of similar appearance in the central part of the breast proved to be benign.

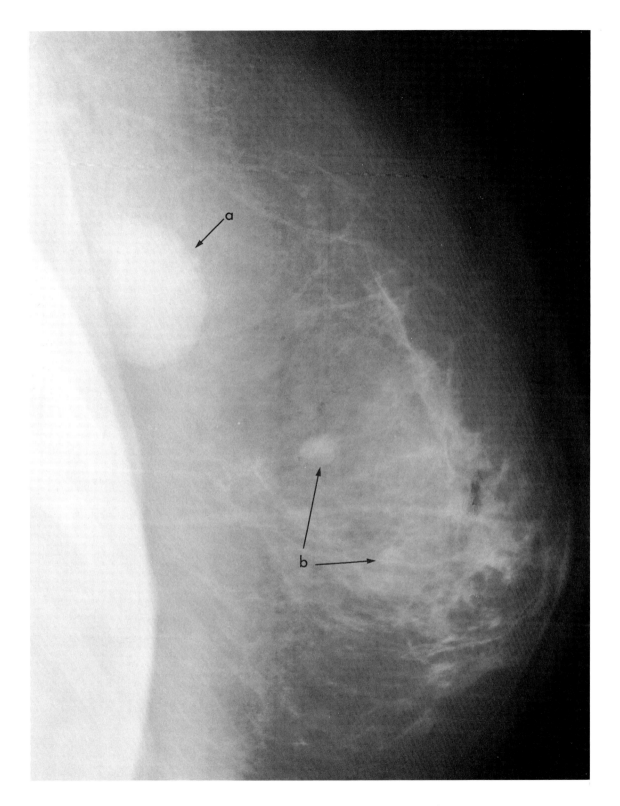

Figure 152 · Rhabdomyosarcoma / 325

Index

CARCINOMA(S) (*cont.*)
  colloid (mucinous), 144, 256–63
    calcification in, 144, 262–63
  diagnosis by
    biopsy, 4
    mammography—accuracy, 2 f.
  infiltrating ductal, with fibrosis, 138
    ff.
  intracystic, 145, 274–77
  lobular, 144, 160–61, 264–69
    calcification in, 144, 264–65,
      268–69
  of male breast, 146, 304–09
  mammary duct ectasia with, 116–17
  medullary, 143, 252–55
  mimicked by
    fibrocystic disease, 49, 82–83
    gynecomastia, 51
    hematoma, 52, 122–23
    herpes zoster, 136–38
    inflammatory diseases, 52 f.
    plasma cell mastitis, 51
    sclerosing adenosis, 49, 88–91
    skin thickening (diffuse), 136
  mimicking benign disease, 139, 160–
    69
  mucinous, *see* Carcinoma, colloid
  multicentric, 145 f., 190–91, 240–
    41, 250–51, 262–63, 268–69,
    282–85
  papillary, 143, 246–51
  during pregnancy, 146, 298–303
    skin thickening in, 146, 302–03
  radiographic signs, 139 ff.
    direct (primary), 139 f., 148–
      89
    indirect (secondary), 140 ff.,
      190–233
  of remaining breast after mastec-
    tomy, 146, 290–97
    new primary, 146, 294–97
  retromammary space obliterated in,
    16
  sclerosing, 138
  scirrhous, 138
    radiographic signs, 139, 148–59
  skin in
    retraction, 141 f., 224–25
    thickening, 141, 172–73, 206–13,
      282–83, 290–91
    ulceration, 142, 226–27

  subareolar, 139, 182–89, 210–11,
    222–23, 250–51
    with comedomastitis, 188–89
    with fibrocystic disease, 184–85
  vascularity increased, 141, 170–71,
    174–75, 214–19
COMEDOCARCINOMA, 142 f., 234–45
  calcification in, 143, 234–35, 238–
    41, 244–45
  infiltrating, 238–45
  noninfiltrating, 234–37
COMEDOMASTITIS, 51, 116–17
  with carcinoma, 188–89
  vs. papillary carcinoma, 143
  and plasma cell mastitis, 51
COMET SIGN: with scirrhous carcinoma, 154–55
CORPUS MAMMAE, *see* Breast, body
CYLINDROMA, 145, 280–81
CYSTOSARCOMA: differentiation from
  cancer, 104
CYSTOSARCOMA PHYLLOIDES, 50, 104–
  107
CYSTS
  see also Fibrocystic Disease
  carcinoma
    beneath, 202–03
    in wall, 145, 274–77
  epidermoid, 126–27
  localized, 47, 54–61
  mimicked by carcinoma, 139, 162–
    63, 166–67
  multifocal, 62–73

F

FAT; FATTY TISSUES
  and age, 17
  postmenopausal, 17, 38–41
  after pregnancy, 17, 32–35
  premenopausal, 17, 36–37
  subcutaneous, 15 f., 20–21, 24–25
  x-ray demonstration, 2
FIBROADENOMA, 49, 96–103
  calcification in, 98–99, 104–105
  giant, 50
  mimicked by
    carcinoma, 139, 168–69
    fibrocystic disease, 82–83
FIBROCYSTIC DISEASE, 47 ff.
  calcifications in, 66–67, 77–83

MENSTRUATION: breast during, 17
MUCIN PRODUCTION: in infiltrative ductal carcinoma, 144

N

NEVUS (OF BREAST), 126–27
NIPPLE(S), 15
bloody discharge in papillary carcinoma, 143, 248
malignant melanoma of, 318–19
normal, 15, 22–23
retraction
in carcinoma, 141, 170–71, 220–23, 258–59, 294–99
congenital, 142, 222–23
skin thickening in Paget's disease, 145, 270–71

P

PAGET'S DISEASE, 144 f., 270–73
PAPILLOMA, INTRADUCTAL, 50, 108–11
with intracystic carcinoma, 274–75
PAPILLOMATOSIS, DUCTAL, 49, 94–95
calcifications as in carcinoma, 141
PREGNANCY
breast in, 17, 42–45, 302–03
carcinoma during, 146, 298–303
fatty breast after, 17, 32–35

R

RADIOGRAPHY OF BREAST, 1 ff.
soft-tissue, 1
RETROMAMMARY SPACE, 16, 20–21
in adolescence, 26
demonstration, 8–9, 18
obliteration
significance, 16
by tumor extension, 142, 228–29
RHABDOMYOSARCOMA, 147, 324–25

S

SARCOMA(S), 147, 318-25
SKIN (BREAST)
benign tumors and tumor-like lesions, 52, 126–27
"dimpling," in carcinoma, 142
retraction in carcinoma, 141 f., 224–25
roentgen demonstration, 15, 22–23
thickening
in carcinoma, 141, 172–73, 206–13, 282–83, 290–91
in carcinoma during pregnancy, 146, 302–03
differentiation, 15
in lymphoma (malignant), 312–13, 316–17
mimicking carcinoma, 136–37
ulceration, in carcinoma, 142, 226–27
SPICULATION: in scirrhous carcinoma, 148–53, 156–59, 214–17
SUBAREOLAR REGION: carcinoma, 139, 182–89, 210–11, 222–23, 250–51

T

TUMORS
benign, 49 ff.
malignant, 138 ff.

V

VEINS (MAMMARY), 16, 20–21, 27
enlargement
with benign lesions, 141
in carcinoma, 141, 170–71, 174–75, 214–20
in menopause, 24–25
in pregnancy, 17, 42–43